1992

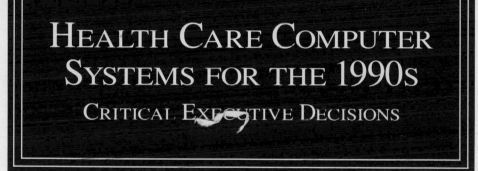

HEALTH CARE COMPUTER SYSTEMS FOR THE 1990s

CRITICAL EXECUTIVE DECISIONS

AMERICAN COLLEGE OF HEALTHCARE EXECUTIVES MANAGEMENT SERIES

Anthony R. Kovner, Series Editor

Bernie Minard

HEALTH CARE COMPUTER SYSTEMS FOR THE 1990s
CRITICAL EXECUTIVE DECISIONS

MANAGEMENT SERIES
American College of Healthcare Executives

95 94 93 92 91   5 4 3 2 1

Library of Congress Cataloging-in-Publication Data

Minard, Bernie.
  Health care computer systems for the 1990s : critical executive decisions / Bernie Minard.
      p.   cm. — (Management series / American College of Healthcare Executives)
    Includes bibliographical references.
    Includes index.
    ISBN 0-910701-67-9 (alk. paper)
    1. Medicine—Data processing.   2. Information storage and retrieval systems—Medical care.   I. Title.   II. Series: Management series (Ann Arbor, Mich.)
    [DNLM: 1. Computers.   2. Health Facilities.   3. Information Systems. WX 26.5 M663h]
R858.M56   1991   362.1′0285—dc20
DNLM/DLC for Library of Congress   90-15620 CIP

The paper used in this publication meets the minimum requirements of American National Standard for Information Sciences—Permanence of Paper for Printed Library Materials, ANSI Z39.48-1984.   ∞ ™

Health Administration Press
A division of the Foundation of the
   American College of Healthcare Executives
1021 East Huron Street
Ann Arbor, Michigan 48104-9990
(313) 764-1380

To my parents, Mary and Ray

CONTENTS

PREFACE

This book is written for executives, managers, and clinical professionals in health care institutions and for students of health care administration. Health care executives are increasingly faced with management issues in the use of information technology as well as opportunities in its effective implementation. Middle-level managers need effective information technology for operation of their departments. Clinical professionals need information technology for storage, organization, and retrieval of data in support of patient care and research. And students of health care administration can benefit from a guide through the bewildering complexity of the issues and options as they begin their careers. Although the focus of the book is on managerial and operational issues in health care, certain relevant modern technological topics are also included.

The purpose of this book is to address these interwoven issues and opportunities and to present strategies and methods that will help health care executives, managers, and clinical professionals to take advantage of this important technology and become competitive leaders in their market segments and fields of professional expertise. Because powerful market forces are pressing hospitals to become full-service health care providers, discussions in this book will use the terms *health care institution* and *hospital* interchangeably to label a modern health care institution of one or more hospitals together with attached or closely linked ambulatory centers, home health care agencies, nursing homes, and physician clinics.

What should health care executives, managers, and clinical professionals expect of information technology and its management in this competitive marketplace? They should expect to use state-of-the-art information technology for competitive advantage. They should expect information technology to be acquired and implemented successfully, remaining flexible to gradual evolution as opportunities are offered by changes in the technology. They should expect the systems and technology to work well when in place. They should expect to have access to powerful data bases that offer easy and responsive access to comprehensive management and clinical information. And they should expect this technology to be managed well, with minimum risk to the institution.

This book covers these expectations. The first chapter, "Health Care and Information Technology: Rapid Change and Growing Opportunities," provides an opening statement about information systems opportunities available to health care institutions. It includes terminology, background and history, an overview of the changing state of the art in information technology and telecommunications, the portfolio of information systems available in health care, recent advances in health care information systems, and the influence of the recent involvement of clinical personnel in clinical information systems.

Chapters 2 and 3 provide an executive guide to planning, management, and control. Chapter 2, "Planning the Information Systems Portfolio," covers planning processes, including variations depending on hospital size and degree of change the hospital is undergoing, how to get started, the importance of linking the information technology plan with the corporate plan, the need to identify strategic systems, the need to involve clinical personnel in planning, and the need to plan an effective portfolio of systems. It includes specific planning methods, illustrations, sample charts and worksheets, planning cycles, and necessary committees and project teams of hospital personnel, including clinical personnel.

Chapter 3, "Organization and Management," focuses on two main themes. The first is the traditional executive management control issue applied to the use of information technology and the challenge of managing limited resources against opportunities that are unclear and changing rapidly. The second theme is the challenge of managing the information services organization, managing the transformation of plans, ideas, and concepts into projects and action. The chapter includes methods and practical aids for executive and managerial control and reporting, project management, change management, problem management, and capacity and utilization management.

Chapters 4 and 5 provide descriptions of two new classes of information technology that are important to health care because they provide the promise of improved productivity through sharing of work and information among the workers of the enterprise. Chapter 4, "Technology: Telecommunications, Networking, and Interconnected Computers," covers the critical and strategic value of data transmission and data networking, the data highways necessary as a foundation for successful use of information technology. It discusses the potential of the technology for health care organizations, recent fundamental changes, terminology, networking objectives, hardware and software, connectivity alternatives, criteria and factors that affect selection, and the management of this technology, including the merging of office automation, telecommunications, and computer technology, and particularly the integration of interconnected, distributed (sometimes called *stand-alone*) islands of computer technology.

Chapter 5, "Technology: Personal Computers and End-User Computing," is the second of the two chapters on information technology. It includes a discussion of end-user computing, the concept of administrative and clinical professionals in hospitals independently using information technology and selected hospital data to do their work. The chapter also includes a discussion of proliferating personal computers and desktop workstations, software and languages, the technology and market, use of the technology by clinical personnel, methods of managing and assuring the value of the investment in this technology, and methods of supporting proficient use of end-user computing.

Chapter 6, "Information Systems Selection and Acquisition," begins a section of two chapters on acquisition and implementation of information systems. Chapter 6 covers the request for proposal (RFP) process, the assessment of current systems and procedures, the definition of required functions and data elements, major types of systems available, evaluation and selection among vendor alternatives, negotiation of vendor assurances in contracts, the concept of life cycles of computer software and hardware, the often overlooked but critical need to be concerned about the integration of and interfacing among systems, and management of the acquisition process. It includes a discussion of the involvement of clinical people (nurses and physicians). It also includes checklists and other aids for managers who have not been through the process before.

Chapter 7, "Systems: Implementation and Institutional Change," shifts to the critical task of managing the teamwork within the diverse groups of people working together on project teams charged with installing the systems, and managing the trauma of organizational change that the new systems and procedures bring. It includes a description of the organization of project teams of clinical, administrative, and information services personnel that must exist during this period, the management of customization of the system, and the comprehensive training and preparation necessary to successfully implement complex new information systems.

Chapter 8, "Protection and Controls for Information Systems Assets: Data Security, Data Integrity, and Disaster Prevention," covers risk and protection. It describes exposures, and evaluation and selection of preventive, detective, and corrective controls against those exposures, including worksheets and an explanation of the analytical risk assessment process that health care executives should undertake. The chapter also describes the requirement for disaster recovery management, the contingency plans for recovering from destruction of the computer center and its contents.

Chapter 9, "The Information Advantage: Managing Data as an Important Resource" focuses on the data stored in the computerized data bases, and the emerging objective of integrating the financial and medical data to the extent that their integration is valuable. It includes a discussion of the concept of storing data in data base management systems (DBMS) and obtaining quick and easy access to that data. It includes discussion of some special data-related problems, such as the overabundance of data, as well as solutions to problems of data integrity and ambiguity, such as those caused by overlapping data timing cycles and the exchanging of data among computers. It also introduces the concept of knowledge-based systems applied to clinical and other hospital data and processes, and the future prospect of using the data bases, together with encoded rules, to mimic the expertise of clinical experts to exploit the data, and to monitor, analyze, and possibly propose action.

Chapter 10, "Looking Ahead: Information Technology and Dramatic Improvements in Health Care," is the final chapter. It looks ahead to the opportunity to use advanced networking technology to do business electronically for improved management and working relationships and productivity across the boundaries of departments, as well as for establishing linkages outside the walls of the health care institution—with physicians, other hospitals, suppliers, and ultimately patients. It explains the potential for integrating medical instrumentation with traditional information systems, including the possibility of transmitting and storing digitized copies of radiology and cardiology diagnostic images. It describes the potential use of information technology at the point of care as a method of capturing more data, relieving nursing people of work, and decreasing the likelihood of data-recording errors. It emphasizes the importance of what is called the computer-human interface, which affects how easy the keyboards, video screens, and pointing devices will be to use. And it stresses the importance of sensitivity to the perceptions of clinical personnel, and the special concern for how clinical personnel will react to a computer information system and, therefore, how quickly the technology will be assimilated and how well it will be used. Finally, it covers advanced issues in managing information technology.

Although knowledge of technical terms is not required to understand the contents of the book, a glossary is included to provide a convenient dictionary of terms that are used in the book, plus some additional terms that are commonly used in the industry.

I wrote this book to provide one central repository for my message that information technology will provide for enhanced productivity and other performance improvements in health care if properly planned and managed. I transferred to the health care industry from another industry because I wanted to solve more meaningful problems. I joined a major hospital that was struggling with a serious management problem. As a very large hospital, it had justified and begun the use of computers early in the computer era, and as later generations of information technology became available, new technology from subsequent eras was acquired and intermixed with that previously installed. Well-intentioned professionals had worked diligently, yet had locked themselves and the hospital into many fragmented and incompatible systems. They had made several management mistakes—poor definition of objectives, poor planning, poor system and technology selection, no hospitalwide executive controls over information technology, and poor management of the work of the computer and other health care professionals—all of which resulted in a confusing maze of poorly functioning systems and islands of technology.

As a result, the hospital was stuck in the midst of several concurrent technological transitions. Technological barriers inhibited further progress toward the completion of system implementations and technological transitions, and other technological barriers prevented a return to an earlier plateau to try another path. In 1980, the hospital still used punched card systems emulating the systems of the 1950s, but it was also naively attempting to use modern telecommunication links among computers and had recently acquired major software tools that it was unable to use effectively. The only path available was to plan very precisely and to use superior management principles, which we did.

Proud of our accomplishment, I wrote articles describing the success of the planning and management principles. Some of the material in this book is adapted from articles that I have written and published in periodicals, including *Computers in Healthcare, Healthcare Computing and Communications, CIO Magazine, Health Care Strategic Management, HealthTexas, Hospital and Health Services Administration,* and *Healthcare Financial Management.* I am grateful for the permissions given by the editors of these periodicals to reuse some of the material in this book.

Neither the book nor the professional and managerial achievements would have occurred, however, without the contributions of the employees and medical staff of The Methodist Hospital in Houston. Above all else, the cooperative work ethic of the managers and other health care professionals throughout the hospital contributed the effort and dedication that made our successes possible. They collectively presented high expectations for themselves and the work of the institution. The employees of the Information Services Division also worked under the high expectations that we set for ourselves, and their competence and dedication led us to the high levels of productivity and quality that we achieved.

I owe many thanks to Donna Falloon, who not only helped type and prepare the several versions of the chapters, but also kept them organized for me. And I am especially grateful to Jennifer Lee and to my wife, Rosemary, who helped enormously in editing the manuscript and offering suggestions.

I am grateful for the contributions of all of these and other colleagues, without whom this book would not have been possible.

1

HEALTH CARE AND INFORMATION TECHNOLOGY: RAPID CHANGE AND GROWING OPPORTUNITIES

The health care business is struggling through a period of fast-paced change in which survival is at stake. Success in this volatile climate depends on nurturing an institutional culture that not only accommodates fast-paced change, but that also uses it to power management processes—processes that enable the institution to seize new opportunities. Information technology offers these opportunities: the possibility of more productive work, more and better access to data, and critical links to off-site relationships.

At the same time, major transformations are also battering the information industry. Explosive technological change is creating new products while making others obsolete, a dramatic evolution that is shaping new methods for planning and managing information technology. Institutions that accommodate this turbulence, successfully planning critical uses of information technology and organizing to manage them well, will ultimately emerge as industry leaders.

Winds of Health Care Change

After years of relative safety, market gluts and competition have finally hit the health care industry—and they have hit it hard. Reductions in government reimbursement for care of Medicare patients, coupled with employers' similar sensitivity to mounting health care costs, have led to lower utilization of inpatient facilities. Patients, too, are shopping around among health care delivery alternatives. The result? Widespread competition among health care institutions.

Though regulation and market changes have been slow to affect health care, they are part of a nationwide trend that has already affected many other industries. Oil companies, airlines, banks, and telecommunications conglomerates, to name a few, have had to meet the challenges of gluts and turbulent market forces with new and creative business techniques.

Now that powerful competitive forces have been unleashed on the health care industry, subtle and comprehensive effects are driving hospitals to change. They will become full-service health care institutions, adding or closely linking themselves with ambulatory care centers and, possibly, home health care agencies, nursing homes, and physician clinics. Those same competitive forces will also drive hospitals into more competitive relationships with other health care providers, suppliers, insurers, employers, and physicians. Consequently, success—and survival—will no longer be as simple and straightforward as it once was.

Like other businesses that are battling market gluts and competition, health care institutions will be forced to focus their efforts on improving productivity. To improve productivity, they will invest money in new information systems, especially clinical systems, that streamline the work processes and logistics with which they deliver services. In this new competitive environment, the very survival of each health care institution is at stake. Some, inevitably, will fall victim to market forces and management challenges. Those that survive will be committed to enhancing clinical work processes and logistics, primarily through creative and effective use of information technology.

However, great barriers must be surmounted in order to reap significant benefits from this technology. Physicians, nurses, and other clinical personnel may not react favorably to the implementation of new information systems in clinical settings. Many factors—the labor-intensive, hands-on nature of health care delivery; the life-or-death consequences of mistakes; the medical and nursing professions' ingrained procedural traditions, personal preferences, and past disappointments with computer technology; society's concerns about the privacy of computerized data; institutions' fear and intolerance of change; and the rapid evolution of information technology itself— will provide major management challenges for institutions that attempt to capitalize on the opportunities provided by information technology.

Evolving Information Technology

The dramatic evolution of the information technology industry spans the past four decades and has involved several major transitions. Computers were first used commercially in the 1950s, when they were purchased for specific single purposes, such as payroll processing. Although single-purpose computers gradually grew larger and evolved to meet several needs, they were still unable to perform more than one job at a time. The payroll department or billing department, for example, shared and scheduled use of the computer when it was not being used by other departments.

The industry underwent its first major transition in 1963 with the advent of IBM's System/360 computer, which offered *multiprogramming,* the capability to process multiple computing tasks simultaneously. This capability gave birth to on-line processing, allowing users remote from the computer center to access the computer through individual video terminals, interrupting the computer from whatever it was processing at the time. This era continued through the late 1960s, when growth in on-line processing strained internal memory capacity limitations in computers. Technology simply failed at that time to provide internal memory management processes sophisticated enough to process simultaneously the growing numbers of on-line transactions.

As the 1970s dawned, another technological breakthrough solved the memory capacity limitation problem. An IBM product, the family of System/370 computers, again had the most publicized effect. It launched the era of high-volume on-line processing. During this era, use of on-line systems in the airlines and brokerage industries burgeoned.

The next transition focused on methods of managing data processing and information systems activities. While information technology provided new capabilities that soon became critical to some industries, sound management principles had not yet emerged to effectively manage either development of required software or its reliable use. During the mid-1970s, top executives pressed for improved management of this important resource, and sound principles, procedures, services, and work-tracking and problem-tracking methods were ultimately forged. During this same period, major software vendors, prompted by similar internal management problems, emerged to provide software packages as a better way to deliver software capability.

A more subtle management transition occurred in the early 1980s. By this time, methods for managing and planning information technology had matured and institutions were beginning to recognize the dependencies between corporate planning and information systems planning. Although institutions were still implementing systems to support their basic business and administration needs, planning efforts began to acknowledge that some systems were more strategic than others. This gave rise to the idea that information systems should be specifically planned, not simply purchased when they became necessary.

At about the same time, personal computers appeared on the scene and were quickly assimilated into the work environment. Mushrooming personal computer usage sparked a need to interconnect personal computers for work and data sharing among people, but information technology vendors, who did not expect the widespread need for networking to arise so quickly, were caught unprepared. As a result, technological support for early networking was weak and lacked the standards necessary to sustain broad, successful usage. Once the value of interconnected personal computers became apparent, however, the great competitive power of this dynamic industry caused a major upheaval in the market for personal computers and networking products, and a steady stream of high-quality products became available.

A great number of useful hardware and software products, such as many word-processing and spreadsheet packages, also evolved during this same period. Unfortunately, each product was created by a different vendor, and each vendor independently designed its own keyboard and video display methods. Although each unique method offered useful and innovative features, the many differences confused users of more than one product and often led to frustration and mistakes. "Exit" and "escape," for example, both emerged as functions that permit users to discontinue a computer process. While the two functions are essentially equivalent, subtle differences do exist in some systems. Even when equivalent, the functions rely on different keys in different systems.

Confusion and frustration resulting from a myriad of these differences gave rise to widespread concern for what came to be called the *computer-human interface,* and demand grew to define universal standards for video and keyboard methods. Consequently, during this transition period, dramatic upheaval occurred in the market for various software products. The methods by which a user interacts with and directs the computer were reconsidered and redefined.

To understand these volatile forces, consider a computer vendor's motivations in the information technology marketplace. Successful vendors must entice customers to buy more and more of their products, so vendors spend their research and development budget dollars on upgrading products' capabilities. Customers who purchase the new and upgraded products embark on a cycle of purchasing advanced products that ultimately leads to technological barriers much like those reached in the early 1960s and 1970s. Vendors then transform the technology and offer new product capabilities that break the barriers. Customers who can economically justify these new capabilities purchase the new products and become early users, paving the way for evolution and later use by other customers.

Currently, the great investment and growth in use of personal computer products have led us to the brink of both a new discontinuity and a new opportunity for breaking barriers in pursuit of interconnectivity and a better computer-human interface. Unlike the past, however, when a few vendors achieved nearly all breakthroughs and advances, today's computer technology market includes many vendors supported by huge investments from suppliers of venture capital. All are competing for market leadership by trying to establish market direction in favor of their product line; all are trying to set de facto standards for the future, also to better position their products. The breakthrough and transition to a new base of products will take several years, but a wide array of partial solutions is already emerging. The challenge to management during this new transition period is to make the right decisions in an era of complex and rapidly changing opportunities. It is a formidable challenge indeed.

Health Care's Use of Information Technology

While businesses in most other industries grew proficient in successfully selecting and using information technology early in its life cycle, health care institutions historically have not been as successful. Information systems projects in health care institutions traditionally were poorly defined and grossly underestimated, and they were invariably oversold—by users who wanted them, by computer systems people who justified their purchase, and by vendors who were marketing their products.

One great inhibitor of effective use of information technology in health care was the nonprofit caretaker attitude that typified the cost-reimbursement era. Few institutions attempted more than a caretaker role, and society apparently did not expect more. Caretaker management simply allowed the complexities of health care to prevent competent use of information technology. For example, the fragmented and ambiguous management structure among medical departments and services, and between the medical staff leadership and hospital administration, offered easy excuses to delay and avoid difficult and uncomfortable computer system activities. On the infrequent occasion when progress was made, it usually came only as the result of a powerful player's special interest, and such successful events were often eventually neutralized: health care institutions simply lacked the management skill necessary to sustain and utilize progress.

Without a strong management structure to plan and define comprehensive and useful information systems, the systems that evolved were weak and fragmented. Major forces driving changes in use of information technology came from outside institutions, in the form of requirements that were defined by government regulations, reimbursement specifications, external auditors' recommendations, physicians' occasional interests, and vendors' marketing efforts.

Reacting to these forces, hospitals installed diverse islands of automation. Large computers (usually called *mainframe computers*) and small computers (usually called *minicomputers*) became fixtures throughout hospitals. The equipment (*hardware*) and computer programs (*software*) came from many vendors; consequently, operating and usage procedures differed widely among the installed systems. These differences were due partly to unique departmental requirements, but some may have resulted from selections calculated to facilitate escape from centralized management influence and control within the hospital.

The resulting collection of information systems was often disparate, disappointing, confusing, and almost impossible to manage. Billing systems frequently used separate and different technology from that of the very registration systems that collected raw billing data. Outpatient registration and billing systems were sometimes incompatible with those used in the very similar inpatient registration processes. The institution's financial accounting system and financial reporting system often used separate and different technology from that of its patient billing systems. Computer systems supporting clinical processes and laboratories were almost always distinct and physically removed from those supporting administrative functions. And, although the industry had high hopes for merging administrative and clinical data from several information systems into a computerized medical record that was to be a cost-effective substitute for voluminous paper processing, that promise was not realized.

Dramatic Changes in Information Systems in Health Care

The regulatory and market influences in health care are changing dramatically, constantly imposing new requirements for information management. In the past, information systems were used primarily for financial and administrative departments, and primarily in support of inpatients. But hospitals are now diversifying into outpatient care and expanding to include several physical facilities, such as ambulatory care centers and long-term care services. These new organizational extensions, together with competitive and cost-control market forces, are requiring executives and managers to embrace information technology as a means to help distribute information among the several health care settings, making integrated patient data available in outpatient as well as inpatient care areas, in remote clinics, in physicians' offices, and in physicians' homes.[1] This new information technology will be expected to improve management of costs, materials logistics, worker productivity, quality standards and controls, and the efficiency of patient care work and scheduling.

Modern information systems will support the simultaneous needs of a variety of health care activities in many departments, whereas information systems designed in the past supported the limited needs of a single department. For example, ADT (admission, discharge, and transfer) systems used in inpatient admitting departments will be replaced by more generalized patient tracking systems that serve both outpatient and inpatient registrations and that distribute work and capabilities beyond the registration departments to nursing and ancillary departments. General ledger systems, previously used only by accounting departments, will be broadened into more general financial reporting systems that provide more information and statistics than just what is necessary to close the books, feeding data directly to department managers and permitting the computerized analytical views of data that are necessary for departmental management and budgeting. Laboratory computer systems will evolve to integrate well with other systems in the health care institution, providing information directly to physicians and nurses in formats relevant to their work. These changes, and the benefits of more efficient integrated computer information systems, will not come easily, and they will require determined and highly competent management.

Past and current industry and market forces are molding the information technology systems and products available to us, few of which are free from significant limitations or are in a form suitable for health care institutions. Following in the next section is a general survey of current and evolving information systems that are available to hospitals, ambulatory centers, and integrated combinations of health care institutions.

Financial and Administrative Information Systems

One of health care management's first objectives is to manage the institution's financial health, an area of major emphasis during the early 1980s as health care providers were faced with dramatic reimbursement changes and diminishing revenues. Consequently, management gave priority to enhanced systems and procedures for patient accounting, receivables management, charge capture, diagnosis-related group (DRG) optimization, claims management, cash posting, management of investments and debt, accounts payable, and managerial control of costs.

Following that, as an extension of cost control, management interest shifted to the more complex management of labor productivity and of materials and supplies. That shift in interest channeled resources into information systems that governed administrative work: patient tracking; room management; order processing; materials acquisition, storage, and flow to work areas; work flow in departments; and tracking of employees' work. These systems improved productivity and efficiency by automating work and reducing manual work loads, transmitting information more quickly and accurately from one work area to another, reducing lost charges, maximizing prospective payment reimbursement, minimizing noncompletion of orders, eliminating duplicate orders, reducing errors, improving quality of patient care by adding controls and exception reports, and, to an extent, using the computer as a Big Brother that monitors and participates in the work of the health care institution.[2] These systems are still evolving, and as they move closer to the work of patient care, they are beginning to resemble the clinical information systems that will likely predominate in the future. Examples of typical financial and administrative systems are described in the following sections.

Conventional financial accounting and reporting

Accounts payable systems automate the paying and recording of invoices and provide controls to prevent mistakes and fraud. Fixed asset systems allow recording of capital assets and their physical location in the institution and also include automated depreciation calculations for proper accounting. General ledger systems provide automated methods of performing formal monthly accounting, including direct entry of journal entries from video terminals. Budgeting systems allow entry and analysis of annual budget data, and integration of that data with general ledger data. Broad financial reporting extensions provide quick ad hoc retrieval of data for analytical purposes, and to spot unusual exceptions or trends, such as displaying a list of all departments that are over budget or that have more than a specific percentage of supplies costs or overtime costs in a given month.

Payroll and human resources management

Employee record keeping is usually consolidated in a system that combines data for payroll, benefits administration, compensation management, employee credentials, and other employee tracking. As in other systems, capabilities are usually included that allow quick ad hoc reporting for special analyses, such as displaying the names of all employees who have licenses, lack required in-services, or have high levels of overtime.

Employee staffing and scheduling

Employee staffing and scheduling systems allow systematic advance scheduling of clinical personnel by day and shift, and sometimes automate payroll time recording as a by-product. Although they sometimes incorporate complex mathematical scheduling, institutions generally find that the mathematical routines of current systems are inflexible and can't meet the changing needs of health care work scheduling. Alternatively, simple record keeping systems that automate the recording of data in rows and columns may be very useful if the data entry and retrieval mechanisms are easy to understand and use. Systems sometimes offer combinations of mathematical optimizations and simple manual scheduling.

Purchasing inventory, materials management, and central supply systems

The logistics of materials are extremely important to health care institutions. Materials management information systems feature records of inventory on hand, reorder levels, order quantities, and usage trends by departments. Charges are automatically created, passed to other systems, and then posted to departments' or patients' accounts. Ordering is usually possible directly from video terminals throughout the hospital. A variety of reports, such as materials usage reports or department usage reports, are available. Newer systems may provide for electronic data interchange (EDI) for automated ordering from vendors, in which case the computer system is connected over telecommunications linkages with the computer systems of major vendors of materials and supplies.

Charge processing, patient accounting, billing, and collections

A master listing of all hospital services and charges is usually administered in a computerized *charge manual*. The computerized charge manual stores and manages charges, descriptions of the charges, and other details, including perhaps work management indicators, such as relative work units (RWU) that indicate work standards for each service. Room rates are also typically included. Computer capabilities provide the means to add or change rates directly from a computer terminal.

The computerized charge manual is part of a comprehensive charge processing, patient accounting, billing, and collections system, the purpose of which is to post daily charges to patients' accounts, screen out errors and display them for correction, issue revenue reports to departments that provide the services, bill patients and other payers, and record payments. The system prorates insurance, automatically produces insurance and other reimbursement claims, and generates patient bills for both inpatient and outpatient services. It also usually produces third-party cost-reimbursement logs, receivables aging reports, collection letters, dunning messages, collection productivity reports, and a broad range of other reports.

Patient identification and tracking, and room and bed management

Comprehensive patient identification and tracking, and room and bed management systems provide for entry and retrieval of data about patients and their locations in the hospital, which help physicians, nurses, blood collectors, and other clinical personnel find patients and provide care efficiently. Such systems support booking and registration of inpatients; emergency room patients; observation patients; outpatients; other institutional patients, such as those being served by home health care activities; and possibly even nonpatients, a situation in which specimens must be analyzed but no actual patient was present. Patient identification data encompass information about insurance, employer, next of kin, and special needs, such as smoking or nonsmoking. Some information specifically related to utilization review and for the purpose of avoiding subsequent denials of payments is also frequently included, such as insurance carriers' specific precertification or recertification requirements. The systems also provide room management capabilities that typically include recording of room conditions, scheduled room cleaning, scheduled patient transfers, room reservations, and real-time recording of patient locations and transfers among the patient rooms and other locations in which patient care is administered. Most systems additionally record data on admitting, attending, and consulting physicians; in such cases the system usually includes information about medical staff privileges, to allow the system to confirm physician admitting privileges. Selected portions of the patient data can be retrieved by many departments, including information desks, physician offices, and patient care departments.

Cost accounting, case analysis, and product line management

Newer information systems dealing with cost accounting, case analysis, and product line management are implemented primarily to provide accurate and timely information to management. Extensions of what were at one time called *case-mix systems* and now often labeled *strategic information systems*, they usually consolidate data from the hospital's charge processing, payroll, materials management, accounts payable, and other transaction processing systems into a data base that also includes work standards for the services provided by each patient care department. Meshed together, these data allow calculation of the cost to provide each service and, therefore, the productivity of each department and the total cost for each patient case, for all cases of a DRG, or for a specific physician's cases. Periodic reports present monthly analyses of both departmental productivity and costs for all patients. Ad hoc displays can be created for special analyses, such as for determining which procedures cause the longest ICU stays or which physicians' patients have the longest length of stay for a given DRG. Modeling of future situations— "what if" analyses of future rate changes, DRG reimbursement changes, or other market-driven changes—could additionally be within the system's capabilities.

Biomedical instrumentation and preventive maintenance recording

Medical equipment and instruments and patient monitoring devices require periodic calibration, checkout, and repair. Computer systems support this function by automatically scheduling necessary maintenance. For example, a specific technician is assigned a computer-generated work list for specific work in a given week, including equipment identification, its physical location, its repair history, and other relevant data. As work is completed, the technician enters into the computer system all details of work performed— details which the technician's supervisor may later display to monitor work status and progress, and equipment condition. Reports can be produced to evaluate technician productivity, repair costs, and other equipment history, or simply to list equipment in the institution.

Physician billing

With physician billing systems, hospitals can provide efficient and cost-effective service to physician groups. These systems post charges (possibly automatically, from data derived from hospital service charges), prepare insurance claims and patient statements, and post payments.

Medical staff record keeping

Medical staff record-keeping systems store and manage data required for periodic credentialing of physicians, including screening of physician privileges when patients register. The scope of physician records encompasses care privileges, dates privileges granted, renewal dates, academic qualifications, licenses, office and home addresses, phone numbers, pager numbers, Medicare provider numbers, and committee assignments.

Risk management and infection control record keeping

A hospitalwide data entry system may be used to collect data about patient falls, medication errors, infections, and other risk management incidents for consolidation into risk management reporting systems. From these data bases, reports on statistics, trends, and other analytical reports can be produced.

Quality assurance record keeping

Quality assurance systems allow entry of data about quality-related incidents, such as occurrence of infection. Quality assurance indicators are usually declared, and periodic reports about incidents and their follow-up by quality assurance personnel are available.

Dietary support

Dietary support systems facilitate menu planning, recipe recording, computation of food ingredients necessary for a given meal, and nutrient planning and analysis. The systems contain data about recipes, menus, inventory, purchase reorder levels, and vendors.

Medical records tracking

Following a patient's discharge, medical records department coders translate data from the patient chart and enter them into a medical records abstracting system that provides a computerized encoded abstract of chart data. Abstracted data elements include diagnosis, disease, treatments, and surgical procedures. Medical records computer systems are also capable of automatically determining appropriate DRGs for Medicare patients, sometimes using algorithms to seek out among allowable alternatives the DRG that produces maximum Medicare reimbursement. These systems can also track completeness of charts by doctor and medical record number or track locations of charts that have been checked out of the department.

Tumor registry

Hospitals must acquire a tumor registry system in order to meet the requirements of professional accreditation agencies. Such systems record details on all tumors diagnosed and treated and are also used to address and compile follow-up letters that are sent periodically to check the status of the patient and the tumor.

Clinical Computer Information Systems

As the capabilities of administrative, logistics, and work management systems are extended to affect work that is increasingly closer to the point of patient care delivery, these systems are becoming the forerunners of the clinical systems of the future. The distinction between conventional financial and administrative systems and systems that directly support clinical processes is eroding and will probably disappear by 1995.[3] For example, cardiology instruments will soon connect directly to cardiology departmental work management and order entry systems, allowing direct transmission of data and even digitized images into computer system files, where mathematical routines may be invoked to help clinicians analyze the data. Such mathematical routines and other knowledge-based system features will permit the system to mimic some of physicians' and technicians' expertise in interpreting data and digitized images. These advanced capabilities will allow the system to combine data from several sources and may lead ultimately to a cost-effective means of producing an all-digital medical record, displacing the paper version of the patient chart.

Clinical information systems potentially can improve the productivity of personnel and the quality of patient care, but these benefits are not automatically realized by all who implement such systems. While clinical information systems promise cost-effective functionality, their early usage has imposed cultural change, complexity, awkward usage procedures, and confusion for physicians and nurses. These users have never really become comfortable with the systems and the technology, and they have reacted negatively to the burdens of technical, procedural, and managerial issues that previously were faced only by information systems personnel. Physicians felt they had not participated in system selection and evolution, that the systems supported clinical processes poorly, and that new capabilities were no better than ordinary manual procedures. They felt that these systems did not add enough value to warrant the investment of effort necessary to master the computerized procedures, and they grew impatient as the slow computer responses could not keep up with their thought processes. Moreover, rapid improvements in computer technology during the recent past led designers to continuously alter and enhance systems. These ever-changing systems, never seemingly completed during long implementation periods, further frustrated clinical users.[4]

Other industries chalked up past successes in many systems projects primarily because computerization elevated, at least temporarily, the new users' status. While these new users in other industries may have been motivated by the excitement of new technology and of gaining special recognition among peers, this is not likely to be a motivating influence on physicians or nurses.[5]

The problems experienced in achieving benefits from clinical information systems are primarily managerial problems, and their solution requires careful management of the involvement of clinical personnel in systems selection, implementation, and usage. Examples of successful clinical systems and uses are described in the following sections.

Order processing

Computerized order processing, the first venture in clinical information system usage, allowed nursing station personnel to transmit electronically physicians' orders to service departments, eliminating both the delays caused by messenger delivery, and the mistakes and missed or duplicated tests that could be caused by faulty manual processes.[6] Moreover, once entered, the orders automatically become computerized work lists for the serving departments, improving management of clinical technicians' work in those departments. Periodic reports of time elapsed between orders and results, along with reports of tests delayed to the following day, also provide an effective tool for productivity assessment and management.

Automatic charge processing is usually a by-product, eliminating possible loss of charges that might for some reason not be entered. Information on order status is another useful by-product. For example, a physician checking the computerized view of the order, and its status, directly from a video terminal at the nursing station or at the physician's office could detect duplicate or incorrect orders. Order entry systems can additionally automatically pass the computerized form of the order and patient identification data directly to clinical laboratory and other departmental systems.

Clinical laboratory

Clinical laboratory computer systems help manage laboratory work by improving productivity and speeding orders through the department. Once an order is entered, either directly from an order entry system or through a video terminal in the laboratory, computer-generated phlebotomist blood collection lists are printed—usually sorted in order by floor and room to boost efficiency by preventing the need to retrace steps. When specimens are collected, each is assigned a sequential number that identifies it during processing by automated lab instruments. As results become available from an instrument, they are passed electronically to the laboratory computer system; manual results are entered through a video terminal. Result verification typically requires a laboratory clinical professional to display the result on a video terminal, verify that it is reasonable and does not require further analysis, and authorize the data for release to others. Clinical laboratory systems sometimes also cover the work management and result-reporting activities of the anatomic pathology department and the blood bank.

Radiology

Like a clinical laboratory system, a radiology computer system provides for improved work management, speeding work through the department and reducing patients' waiting time. Patient identification data and orders are frequently received directly from the order entry system, but they may also be entered manually into the radiology computer system. Orders are compiled into work lists and assigned to technicians, equipment and rooms are assigned (in some systems, patient appointments are scheduled), and the films are taken. These films are interpreted, comments are dictated, and word-processing clerks transcribe the dictated results into the computer system, often retrieving paragraphs of prestored text to describe normal results. The system is additionally used to track the location of radiology films.

Radiology systems can reduce lost charges, improve accuracy of charges, reduce patients' waiting time, improve departmental productivity, speed results to nurses and physicians, and prevent duplicate tests. Advanced systems may also provide a means for digitizing radiology images and transmitting, storing, and displaying them on high-resolution computer screens at locations other than where the film is located, such as directly at a nursing station. These systems may also offer digitized voice-recording capabilities, eliminating the need for dictation equipment by storing the radiologist's comments in the computer files along with digitized film and text data.

Pharmacy

Pharmacy computer systems simplify and streamline medication dispensing and inventory control. Computerized records for each active inpatient and outpatient contain patient identification data, age, sex, diagnosis, allergies, drug sensitivities, and the profile of all medications taken during the current episode of illness. Records for each drug include identification, cost, charge, amount on hand, order quantities, and related inventory data. These systems automate production of medication labels and daily refills of patient orders, and even reorder from the distributors. Modern pharmacy systems also automatically check all drug orders and dosages against patients' allergies, other drugs being taken, and diet orders, possibly preventing delivery of medications that could be harmful.

Cardiology

Cardiology department computer systems, like radiology department computer systems, help manage departmental work and also provide printed and electronic results to other clinical personnel. Patient identification information and orders may either be received automatically from an order entry system or entered manually, while results are usually entered manually from the several cardiology department sections. The system organizes and formats data; presents the data on reports for distribution to cardiologists, surgeons, other physicians, and nurses; and may also electronically transmit computerized variations of the reports for display at nursing stations and physicians' offices. Work load statistics reports are often available for department managers, and retained patient data can be used for research purposes. Additional system features can include inventory management for high-cost critical items like catheters. Advanced systems may allow digitized images to be collected directly from cardiology diagnostic equipment, stored, transmitted, and later retrieved along with text reports.

Pulmonary function and respiratory therapy

Pulmonary function and respiratory therapy computer systems typically are connected to instruments that automatically collect patient data regarding respiratory flow rate and lung capacity. They employ mathematical calculations to analyze and graph that data, compare them to norms, and allow interpretation by pulmonary specialists, who may use the system's word-processing capabilities to present text interpretations for ordering physicians. These text interpretations can then be passed automatically to results retrieval systems for display at nursing stations and physicians' offices. Respiratory therapy management may be part of the same system or provided by a separate system. As in other clinical systems, orders and patient identification data may come from an order entry system. Management statistics reports are also usually available, such as therapists' workload efficiency reports and reports on responsiveness and delays in servicing orders.

Radiotherapy

Radiotherapy department computer systems, similar to other departmental systems, feature capabilities for accepting patient identification and patient orders directly from order entry systems, formatting those orders to become work lists for department personnel and compiling work management statistics as a by-product. Advanced systems provide powerful computerized mathematical routines that present three-dimensional images on video displays for physicians and radiotherapy technicians who are planning patient treatments.

Results retrieval

When tests and treatments are completed and entered into the computer system in ancillary departments, computerized forms of the numerical and text results are stored in data bases and are available at video terminals in nursing stations, physicians' offices, and other authorized locations. To protect vital data confidentiality, these systems should provide a means to limit the display to only those authorized, and only at locations where patient care is given. For example, results may be displayable at physicians' offices, but only at those of the attending physician or other physicians associated with the case. Personnel at nursing stations might have access only to data concerning patients physically present on that unit. Results should be selectable by time and type (for example, all chemistry results during the past 24 hours) and also available for optional printing at adjacent printers. Advanced systems present numerical test data in flowcharts and in graphic form, both on the video display and on the printers, and also display digitized images directly at nursing station and physician office terminals. Advanced systems may also scan for combinations of conditions that may alert clinicians to problems, or otherwise help clinicians enhance the quality of care provided to patients.

The computerized patient chart or computerized medical record

Because results retrieval computer systems collect a large portion of the information that is also printed in paper form and stored in patient charts, it seems logical to expect that these results will eventually be consolidated and stored in computerized files, becoming the computerized medical record of the future. But, although some progress toward this end has been made, problems have plagued efforts to collect the accurate, consistent data required and to structure the data for subsequent retrieval.[7] These problems arise because patient chart data are produced by a wide variety of departments and people, with accuracy and consistency depending on many sources. The data must further be transformed into electronically readable and structurable form. Only a small portion of the raw data—essentially, the results of tests and procedures—is likely to take that form, and even these data are usually generated by several vendors' systems and, therefore, are likely to be in different formats. The remainder of the data (handwritten progress notes, graphs, tables of rows and columns of data, or images) must be transformed into digitized form. To integrate these data, patient, date, and other codes must be added so that the system can identify and retrieve the records for later use.

As technology advances and more data are computerized, such as nursing notes, vital signs, and medications administered, some of these problems will be resolved. These advances, combined with continued improvement in physicians' and nurses' skills with, and acceptance of, computerized medical data, will lead to wider use of large clinical data bases and, ultimately, to a computerized medical record and potentially improved patient care outcomes.

Operating room management and scheduling

Operating room management systems facilitate efficient scheduling, reduce clerical work requirements and improve accuracy in the operating room log, and reduce work and improve accuracy in patient charges. When data required to maintain the operating room log are entered into the system, reports on utilization and turnaround of operating room suites are typically generated for management analysis as a by-product. Scheduling of surgical cases is usually provided, both for individual cases and by block. In advanced systems, materials requirements planning and physician preference checklists allow the system to display or report the materials and supplies necessary to prepare for specific surgical procedures. Following surgery, this computerized materials and supplies list is amended based on actual usage, and the operating room suite times are entered as part of the log, allowing patient charges to be automatically passed to the patient accounting system for posting.

Patient appointment scheduling

These systems allow scheduling of patients for tests and treatments within the health care institution, and possibly for related visits to physicians' offices when they are physically adjacent. It may serve inpatients or outpatients exclusively, or in a modern hospital with high-volume ambulatory care services, it may serve both. Such a system is particularly useful now, when more and more tests and treatments that were once performed in an inpatient setting are instead performed in an outpatient setting. In fact, it may not be possible to provide effectively such outpatient services without an efficient scheduling system that coordinates the work of physicians, physicians' office staffs, and hospital nursing and ancillary department personnel. Scheduling systems reduce patient waiting time, improve efficiency of hospital personnel, reduce staffing needs (which may decrease when work is scheduled), and possibly automate charge capture, thereby reducing lost charges.

Nursing support systems in intensive care and general care units

Nursing support systems, the most recent advances in computer systems for health care, reduce the quantity and improve the accuracy of nursing paperwork, such as nursing care planning, recording of vital signs, and nursing notes. By making data easier to record and retrieve, these systems may also reduce the time and cost spent on those tasks. Nursing support systems partition documentation into its components, such as nursing diagnosis and nursing interventions, and staff members typically enter data with a keyboard or by using screen pointing tools to select from a menu of choices on a video screen.

Bedside and portable data collection devices have also recently become available, allowing nurses to enter medication administration data using bar codes and to enter vital signs directly from digitized instruments at the bedside. With this new technology, other nursing data can additionally be captured and entered directly at the patient's bedside, potentially improving both productivity and the accuracy of charting.[8] In intensive care units, patient monitoring equipment is connected directly into the nursing support system, allowing automatic entry of physiologic data, such as blood pressures and cardiac rates, and automating the flow sheet.

Nursing support systems also feature patient classification capabilities so that nurses can enter ratings for a number of work intensity indicators, such as whether or not a patient must be fed or can feed himself or herself. These indicators are aggregated and transformed into a patient acuity score for each patient, and the system calculates the nurse staffing requirements for that nursing unit. Nursing support systems can also offer severity-of-illness capabilities, which allow nurses to enter clinical data about the patient's illness severity or disease stage. With this data, the intensity and criticality of nursing work can be measured, and trends can be analyzed.

Messaging and information distribution

Hospital information systems frequently incorporate messaging systems that allow some forms of electronic messaging and information transmission. Electronic mail capabilities allow users to send messages much as they would telexes. A message is composed at a video terminal and then directed to one or more specific workstations or persons. If the message is sent to a workstation, it is displayed immediately when the receiving terminal is on-line; when the receiving terminal is not on-line, the message is displayed as soon as it does come on-line. If the message is sent to a person, the system uses the concept of an electronic mailbox, where the message waits until the person signs on and, informed that mail exists, retrieves it. In systems used widely by physicians and other clinicians, messages related to a consultation or other patient care matters can be sent from one physician's office to another.

Beyond messaging, these systems also typically allow routine distribution of schedules, announcements, or notices about new system functions and training sessions. Advanced systems can distribute medical information such as protocols for the determination of death or limitation of treatment, as well as text data such as medical staff bylaws.

Systems for support of medical decisions

Experimental systems developed in the academic medicine environment attempt to assist in the diagnosis of illness. These systems, often called *knowledge-based* or *expert systems,* contain large numbers of embedded rules and data. Although they are useful in teaching, especially within narrow subfields of medicine, such systems seldom assimilate enough information to be useful clinically. These systems are undergoing constant expansion, however, and continuing advances may justify wider application in the future.

Options for Acquisition and Management of Information Systems

The market provides several options for acquiring computer hardware and software. A hospital may acquire both hardware and software from a single vendor in what often is called a *turnkey* contract, under which the vendor completely implements the system and then turns the key over to the hospital to manage the system's use. The same vendor typically provides all future hardware and software upgrades in the same turnkey manner and also usually contracts to perform all problem solving and software corrections when difficulties are discovered. The hospital may acquire several different turnkey systems from several vendors, but all must operate in concert to meet the hospital's needs.

In an alternative strategy, the hospital may acquire computer hardware from a vendor while reducing operational complexity by running several software systems on the one computer. This approach offers the option of acquiring systems either all at once or separately over a period of time. As another variation, the hospital may acquire hardware and software and then use its own programming staff to develop additional software.

On the other hand, a hospital could gain access to computers located elsewhere, arranging to have some or all of its information systems operated on that computer and some or all of its video terminals connected to the distant computer. For example, a public hospital could use city or county computer facilities, a hospital in a multihospital system might share the corporate computer center, or a university hospital may use the university's computer center.

In a variation on this theme, some vendors provide hospitals with access to information systems operating on computers located at the vendor's site, where usage is shared among many hospitals. For example, payroll data or patient charge data collected throughout the day at the hospital may then be transmitted to the vendor for processing; the resulting computer reports are transmitted electronically or mailed back to the hospital the following day. Video terminals in the hospital connect to this distant computer for entry and retrieval of data.

However, as computers have become smaller, less expensive, and easier to use, many hospitals that previously used vendors' or other entities' shared systems are now electing to discontinue prior arrangements and gradually acquire their own on-site computer systems. Such acquisition sometimes begins with a personal computer system or other small computer system that offers capability not provided by the distant system. The small in-house computer system frequently is then extended for use by several people or several departments through use of local area networks. Other similar small systems that eventually are acquired are similarly extended, and then the several systems are interconnected, also using local area networking. Ultimately, the hospital accumulates a core of systems—and enough confidence with use of this new technology—to lead them in planning and gradually acquiring an integrated set of on-site information systems.

Vendors also offer facilities management contracts, an arrangement in which a vendor manages a computer system on the hospital's premises. For example, a hospital that acquires a computer system may not initially possess the expertise necessary to manage the facility. One solution is to contract for several years of facilities management service, either from the vendor of the system or from another firm specializing in facilities management services.

When an institution chooses to combine these alternatives, the resulting simultaneous use and management of several different systems can present formidable challenges. For example, systems that operate on varying computer models could force users to learn different software terminologies and computer control statements. Additionally, some systems may be at the hospital and some at the vendor's site, with possibly one or more being operated under a facilities management contract. Each system requires users to develop proficiency with a different set of skills, making usage more difficult and less accurate as users confuse methods of one system with those of another. Similarly, each system calls for different operations management skills. Finally, a mixture of several options can make systems interconnection and data integration extremely difficult to achieve.

Integration and Interconnection

When management directed that islands of automation throughout the hospital be interconnected to exchange data, transition to a new era began. The requisite first step focused on a difficult task: providing a physical connection and method of exchanging data among computers, called a *computer interface*. The computer interface requirement varied among institutions and situations, but the solution was almost invariably complex. Early interfaces were generally unreliable and unpredictable, with few controls to ensure that all required exchanges occurred without loss, redundancy, and ambiguity. Technological details of the interface were difficult to comprehend, and procedures were poorly defined and intricate.

Today, providing high-quality computer interfaces among systems is still a challenging issue that merits significant management attention when planning and installing health care information systems. Computer interfaces are discussed in detail in Chapter 6.

The Need for Sound Knowledge

Ironically, many of today's health care executives and professionals reached their current positions before information technology became a vital part of health care delivery. Similarly, many managers in information technology departments were promoted from lower-level data-processing positions before information technology assumed its current level of importance. Consequently, they often lack business, management, and leadership skills necessary to manage the information technology on which the institution depends. Some institutions, therefore, have the worst possible combination. They are led by executives who are uneasy with the terminology, concepts, and decisions of information technology, who associate computers with the basement, and who retain the fairly low opinions they formed of earlier computer systems and the data-processing people who operated them. At the same time, these institutions employ information technology managers who, in fact, previously performed data-processing tasks on those same basement computers.

Successful executives, managers, and health care professionals of the future will be equipped to make intelligent information technology decisions without discomfort or hesitation. Additionally, the person who assumes responsibility for the information systems function must possess leadership skills and business acumen far beyond the scope of traditional data processing.

Today's Information Technologies: Merging and Changing

Computer technology has changed dramatically. Personal computers, already quite useful in health care institutions, become even more valuable when they successfully function together on networks. Data communications technology has revolutionized the telecommunications industry, providing a wealth of new opportunities. The reliability of hardware and, to a lesser extent, software have improved significantly. The once-sharp lines between computing, office automation, and telecommunications technologies are blurring and overlapping. In fact, they could essentially be aggregated as providers of a cluster of capabilities labeled "information technology."

As defined earlier, computer equipment is called *hardware* and computer programs are called *software*. For management purposes, the distinction is necessary only because hardware is typically purchased or leased while software is, instead, licensed. Software that is almost indistinguishable from hardware, called *system software,* is usually licensed from the hardware vendor. For example, personal computer software called DOS (an acronym for Disk Operating System) is system software. This system software, frequently referred to as *operating system software,* enables the computer to function as a computer.

The other type of software, which provides automation for defined business functions like patient billing, is called *application software.* So named because the resulting computerized work is an "application" of computer use, this software is typically provided by many vendors, including some that also market hardware.

Current leading-edge improvements in hardware capability center on the decreasing size of electronic components. The same phenomenon sparked sweeping changes in home entertainment appliances: vacuum tubes were first replaced by transistors and then by etched deposits on silicon chips smaller than coins. New, smaller components require less electric power, emit less heat, are more reliable, and can be placed closer together, allowing electrons to reach their destinations by traveling over shorter distances and, therefore, operating at faster speeds. A recently manufactured computer or piece of computer equipment consequently costs less and fails less often than those of earlier generations.

As component sizes reach their lowest limits, focus will shift to other technological directions in ongoing efforts to increase the speed of computers. New and future technology will harness many computer processing units together in tandem so that they appear to be, and function as, one computer.

The resulting new capability will expand the computer's power to handle larger volumes of transactions and larger computing loads. This symbiotic approach, known as *parallel processing,* is part of a technological transition that will also require evolution to complex systems software. Future software will organize and partition the computer's work so that it is assigned to many internal computer units for simultaneous processing. Advancements in parallel processing computer technology will likely provide the breakthrough that allows powerful future computer systems to support computer technology at the patient's bedside and in increasingly sophisticated patient monitoring systems.

Future enhancements in computer software will be sustained by computer scientists' dramatic continuing work in universities and private corporations, just as any other field of science grows as continuous research and development contribute to the body of scientific knowledge. At an earlier time, the industry could not invest effort in improving the functionality of operating systems, both because many hardware and software capabilities had not yet emerged and because all available computer system design and computer programming resources were required to keep systems functioning reliably at their early design levels. Today, however, system software is being enhanced to provide more functions, such as managing the simultaneous processing of several computers within one computer or performing automated self-diagnosis of functions in hardware—and even in the software itself. Existing application software is being improved to provide more reliable and richer functions. New application software is being written to expand functions beyond the processing of existing business transactions, providing systems that, for example, make it easier to access and analyze data or to simulate the work of experts. Currently, the technological capabilities that are changing most rapidly and dramatically are the speed and telecommunications method of data transmission. Terminology and changing directions related to these capabilities are examined in Chapter 4.

The three interdependent technological capabilities—computer hardware technology, systems software, and data networking—are usually referred to collectively, using a single term. *Technological platform* is one such term, but other synonymous terms are also used: *technological infrastructure, technological architecture,* and *underlying architecture.* An institution's technological platform is crucial because it determines which computer applications may be feasible at the institution. A weak, poorly planned, poorly implemented technological platform severely limits computer applications that the institution may install.

It is therefore vital that institutions plan their technological platform carefully and manage it well. All three capabilities must evolve together, prudently incorporating changes in a choreographed sequence that projects two or more years into the future. Computer technology functions in any of the three capabilities are prerequisites of functions in the other two. If managed poorly, technological advances easily available to others may be impossible or require years to implement—while aggregate capabilities may function unreliably and problems may defy diagnosis.

On the other hand, institutions that effectively manage their technological platform will keep pace with evolving technology, reaping the rich rewards of both compatibility among information technology products and flexibility to meet future requirements.

Notes

1. M. A. Daniels et al., "Patient Care Information Systems in a Diversified Environment," *Topics in Health Care Financing* 14, no. 2 (Winter 1987): 36–37.
2. R. M. Sneider, *Management Guide to Health Care Information Systems* (Rockville, MD: Aspen Publishers, 1987), pp. 161–68.
3. H. H. Schmitz, *Managing Health Care Information Resources* (Rockville, MD: Aspen Publishers, 1987), p. xiv.
4. J. G. Anderson and S. J. Jay, "The Diffusion of Computer Applications in Medical Settings," in *Use and Impact of Computers in Clinical Medicine,* ed. J. G. Anderson and S. J. Jay (New York: Springer-Verlag, 1987), pp. 3–7.
5. D. W. Young, "What Makes Doctors Use Computers?: Discussion Paper," in *Use and Impact of Computers in Clinical Medicine,* ed. J. G. Anderson and S. J. Jay (New York: Springer-Verlag, 1987), pp. 8–14.
6. W. P. Pierskalla and D. Woods, "Computers in Hospital Management and Improvements in Patient Care—New Trends in the United States," *Journal of Medical Systems* 12, no. 6 (1988): 412.
7. Q. E. Whiting-O'Keefe et al., "The STOR Clinical Information System," *M.D. Computing* 5, no. 5 (September/October 1988): 8–20.
8. M. A. Stefanchik and P. I. Cohen, "Point-of-Care Faces Cost Challenges," *Computers in Healthcare* (December 1989): 38–39, 41.

2

PLANNING THE INFORMATION
SYSTEMS PORTFOLIO

The earliest era of computer usage was relatively simple and compartmental-ized; therefore, it sparked little serious concern for planning information technology. As businesses and computers evolved, however, increased op-portunities for the use of information technology and greater dependence on that technology forced management to acknowledge planning as a necessary function. Eventually, a few, generally larger, health care institutions found value in planning and incorporated it as an essential and regular part of their management practices. Other institutions, however, which found planning less valuable, simply went through the motions, perfunctorily and irregu-larly, or avoided it altogether.

In spite of the current abundance of published information about plan-ning and its acceptance as a necessary routine, planning is still often reduced to little more than a list-making exercise. All too often, it is thought to be trivial and disappointing, and an unimportant high-level management respon-sibility. Rarely is it regarded as the valuable activity that it can be.

The question remains: Is planning information technology really so important? Why not just respond managerially when operational problems or other management issues arise? Why plan?

Pressures to Plan

Pressures to plan come from many sources.[1] For example, management's frustration with continuing information technology problems creates pres-sures to plan, as does the desire to avoid frequent costly waves of technologi-cal upgrade and replacement. Another source of planning pressure is management's realization that unwise use of information technology could cost the institution valuable competitive opportunities. Management may simply sense that its corporate strategic plan depends heavily on successful use of information technology.

As planning pressures grow, planning for information technology evolves through developmental phases, from short term and simple to long term and complex. Generally, these phases appear in larger health care institutions before they appear in institutions that are smaller, less complex, and less affected by the frustrations of problems and lost opportunities due to a poor fit of information technology to their needs. During the early phases of evolution of an institution's information technology, incentives to plan are usually the result of pressures to solve specific problems that management has deemed critical. In this early phase, both large and small health care institutions are generally limited in their understanding of information technology and, therefore, limited in their ability to develop long-term plans for their use. Planning, therefore, is of a short-term nature and focused on finding solutions to individual problems.

Successful short-term planning during this early phase, however, builds understanding and confidence that lead gradually to a more sophisticated use of planning. During this second phase, planning for upgraded resources becomes more detailed, and priorities are established for longer-term projects. Planning in this second phase also includes assessment of current work and provides project lists and time schedules for acquiring information technology resources and implementing information systems. However, because institutional goals change and institutional understanding of the technology changes, these lists and schedules may ultimately not be strictly followed.

The use of computer information systems planned during the second phase, combined with management's growing understanding of computers, will generate new pressures to enhance systems during an evolving third phase. Planning pressures during this third phase will center on upgrading the recently installed systems to improve managerial controls, efficiency, and productivity, and to solve problems caused by the introduction of new information systems during the second phase.

The successful planning of the third phase will provide momentum that will lead to a fourth phase in which pressures shift to plan for information technology to cover a longer time period. In this phase, the institution will plan for a wider spectrum of systems, to make use of information technology to increase its competitive advantage.

Although the four planning phases may occur sequentially, as described above, an institution's planning process may be made more complex by the simultaneous presence of pressures from several or all phases, especially as computer technology, office automation, and telecommunications merge to provide important collective capabilities. During the evolution and maturation of an institution's use of information technology, these many planning pressures shift—and the objectives and value of planning shift with them. So, although one planning objective may be fully served during an early phase, continuous, comprehensive long-range planning is still important for other reasons. Throughout all phases, the institution must continue to plan improvements and additions that will prolong the life and usefulness of systems. Otherwise, systems may require premature replacement, which, of course, is costly and inefficient.

In many health care institutions, both large and small, the planning process may become progressively more complex and difficult. As unforeseen early problems and later opportunities are identified, and planning pressures shift as planning phases evolve, early plans are invalidated and will have to be reconsidered and updated. As a result, confidence in the plan and the planning philosophy may weaken. Under such conditions, formulating a sound plan for guiding the institution through a transformation is very difficult and requires strong executive leadership.

Today's era of high expectations for information technology is not only driven by a computer-literate work force and intensive marketing of information technology, but also inhibited by limited corporate resources and ambiguity in the computer technology marketplace. In this uncertain environment, how does management set priorities for computer projects in which to invest the institution's resources? Furthermore, why is it more difficult in health care to plan the optimum portfolio of information systems?

The Challenge of Planning Health Care Information Systems

Several issues unique to the health care industry make planning and implementing information systems a difficult and complex process. To begin with, health care decisions have a direct—and critical—effect on the lives of patients.[2] Planning under these conditions, therefore, takes on an element of urgency, and alternatives require painstaking analysis before decisions are reached.

Health care information systems also potentially replace detailed, time-honored record-keeping systems that are virtually embedded in the nursing and medical professions. Consequently, potential changes brought by automation require agonizing scrutiny to make certain that they are acceptable before agreements to change them can be reached.

Furthermore, data confidentiality is far more important in health care than in any other industry. At the same time, however, data stored in hospital information systems can be extremely important to patient care and should, therefore, be on-line and available for immediate inquiry throughout the hospital. These conflicting requirements for both confidentiality and accessibility of patient information necessitate planning for intricate controls and special procedures through the computer information system.

Implementing a computer information system in any institution is an integrating process that mingles the tasks and responsibilities of different employees. In most businesses, these employees make up a fairly homogeneous work force. Health care institutions, however, must invest significant time and energy integrating the work of several different employee populations, leading the various and differing populations to an understanding of, and agreement on, the integrating effect of changes that automation may bring.

Finally, the health care industry has a high percentage of professionals in various decision-making positions. These professionals, principally clinical professionals, who are selected to serve on medical, nursing, and other professional staffs because management respects their knowledge and skills, naturally expect to influence decisions, and their contributions are exceedingly valuable. At the same time, it is important to recognize that they often may represent conflicting spheres of interest within the institution. The challenge to health care management, therefore, is to include clinical and other professionals in information systems planning without allowing the needs of any particular interest group to prevail at the expense of others.

What to Plan: Selecting One Information Systems Project over Another

The array of opportunities for using information technology in an institution is often so great that no clear direction is immediately apparent. Information technology targeted for already exemplary departments or activities may make them stronger. Alternatively, targeting information technology for areas that obviously need help may spark their turnaround.

How should management choose among alternatives for investment of information systems resources? Should traditional economic justification serve as the principal guide? Should planning methods or criteria be different in large and small health care institutions? Are there other important considerations? In general, how should information systems projects be planned?

Systems Concepts and Definition of a System

The term *system* is in wide use, since systems concepts provide a useful framework for labeling organized arrangements of processes. Concepts from general systems theory are used to describe and understand many processes in many disciplines, including decision making and control in health care institutions.[3] General systems theory concepts are applicable also to use of the term *information systems*.

In the theory, a system is a set of elements that operate together to accomplish an objective, as in a freeway system, a school system, or a group of hospitals and other health care institutions operating together as a system. A system requires three essential elements: input, an internal process, and output. Systems have boundaries, beyond which other systems may function, and possibly interconnect. Interconnected systems are also termed *systems*, causing the term *subsystem* to be used to label a system within a system. Consequently, since most systems function as part of a greater system, the two terms *system* and *subsystem* are used synonymously.

An institution generally labels its information systems based on their support for major institutional processes, such as a financial accounting system, an order entry system, or a clinical laboratory system. These systems are really hierarchies, or other interconnected linkages, of many basic subsystems. Some of the subsystems are manual subsystems and some are computer-based subsystems. Moreover, both the manual and computer-based subsystems are interconnected linkages of more basic subsystems. Subsystems at the most basic level accept input, process it, and produce output.

Starting the Planning Process: An Assessment

For the hospital, large or small, that has never planned its information systems before, the planning process begins with a straightforward assessment of current systems and problems. The initial step in the first planning phase requires the institution to compile a complete inventory of all the institution's currently functioning information systems, as shown in Exhibit 2.1. This inventory provides a listing of the hospital's current portfolio of information systems. At the same time, a complete inventory of all incomplete information systems projects, both under way and planned, must also be compiled. This listing should include descriptive information, as shown in Exhibit 2.2.

Together, these two lists form the foundation for detailed record keeping that will be used first for the initial assessment and later for planning the future portfolio. Moreover, such record keeping, continued throughout

Exhibit 2.1   An Example of a Complete Inventory of an Institution's
Information Systems

Current Portfolio of Information Systems
As of May 1, 1989

System	Manager Responsible
Biweekly payroll system	Smith
Monthly payroll system	Smith
General ledger and financial reporting system	Jones
Accounts payable system	Jones
Patient registration system—inpatients	Doe
Patient registration system—outpatients	Doe
Accounts receivable system—inpatients	Doe
Accounts receivable system—outpatients	Doe
Pathology department system	Brown
Radiology department system	Brown
Order entry at nursing stations	Brown
Operating room log (personal computer) system	Black
Medical staff office physician recordkeeping system	Black

Exhibit 2.2   An Example of an Inventory of Incomplete Information
Systems Projects

Computer Systems Projects Underway
As of May 1, 1989

Project Description	Department Requesting	Current Status	Remaining Staff-Days
Enhance patient registration and accounts receivable systems to provide special handling codes for each patient	Patient accounting	Complete, awaiting acceptance	0
Enhance human resources system to allow printing of comprehensive annual benefits statements	CEO	Testing under way	5
Enhance patient tracking system to allow charging for room overtime for medical necessity or patient convenience when appropriate	Business office	Programming under way, scheduled for first use July 1	15

system installation and planning, also provides an accounting of the work effort invested in each system—data that may ultimately be used in planning upgrades or eventually replacing the systems.

Planning Initial Systems Activities that Will Reduce Problems

An evaluation of each current system and project under way enables management to assess the approximate number of staff-hours of effort being expended in support of each system and project. Once these approximations are calculated and ranked, the systems with the highest level of effort should be examined closely, because a high level of effort spent maintaining and remedying problems for any system in the institution's current portfolio usually signals a major problem. Perhaps the system fails frequently, causing problems for employees and others throughout the institution. Or perhaps the high level of effort may exist because the system is used inappropriately or because system users are improperly trained and depend heavily on assistance from information systems employees to recover from problems that could have been avoided with adequate training. Excessive levels of effort may even signal shortcomings within the information systems group: for example, information services personnel may not be properly installing high-quality systems or may lack competence in maintaining them. Persistently high work levels for maintaining systems usually indicate problems either in the management of the information systems department or in the departments that the systems serve.

There are exceptions, however, and high levels of maintenance do not always signal such major problems. Newly installed systems usually require extra maintenance simply because they are new both to information systems personnel and to users. New systems usually have marginal controls and greater opportunity for errors, flaws, oversights, and mistakes by unfamiliar users. Replacement systems offer a similar, but smaller, risk of high maintenance levels.

System enhancements, on the other hand, generate far fewer errors and problems and do not usually contribute to a major increase in maintenance when they are installed. Because system enhancements change work that is already familiar to the work force, proposals for enhancements usually anticipate and prevent major problems. This observation leads to a valuable basic strategy. Planning the installation of systems in steps, with the simplest base installed initially and other functions added gradually as necessary and when personnel have mastered the latest enhancements, is a sound strategy that minimizes operational problems and maintenance work.

Planning Systems that Support Institutional Objectives

A sound information technology plan is guided by the hospital's long-term objectives. Details of the corporate plan provide assistance in selecting among the myriad opportunities for information systems that are required to support the business. However, even after systems are selected to support the institution's objectives, the planning process should provide for a periodic cycle of reevaluation and revision of the corporate plan to reflect a continuously changing business climate. In hospitals that use this methodology,[4,5] as the corporate plan evolves, so does the information technology plan. Also, periodic reevaluations will determine if new and emerging technology could serve the corporate plan's goals and objectives better than technology previously planned.

In addition to an evolving corporate plan, the changing opportunities offered by information technology itself pose an additional challenge to the planning process. Because these evolving opportunities might offer new business alternatives that could affect it, the corporate plan must be reevaluated in light of emerging information technology possibilities. Consequently, the corporate plan and the information technology plan are linked symbiotically, with neither subordinated to the other.

Planning New Information Systems

A modern hospital is an information-intensive institution that must continuously invest its resources in new and replacement information systems. Without such ongoing investment, the institution risks facing a future operational crisis created by an entire portfolio of obsolete systems that would have to be completely replaced over a short time span. Moreover, by continuously adding new and replacement systems, the hospital ensures that new processes are automated and, therefore, new data items are collected and stored, thereby contributing to the data bases of accurate, up-to-date information that are indispensable to successful operation.

Planning Projects that Provide a Sound Return on Investment

Information systems may provide value in reducing costs or increasing profitability and, therefore, provide a sound financial return on the investment. If the return on investment is higher than the cost of financing available, the project qualifies for approval.

Planning System Enhancements

System enhancements usually offer the best return on investment among information systems opportunities. Users base their proposals for enhancements on sound knowledge of existing systems and procedures, and this familiarity usually results in proposals that accurately anticipate both the value of enhancements and the difficulty of accompanying problems. Furthermore, strong institutions that invest in their established areas of strength generally succeed in making themselves even stronger. Together, these arguments make a strong case for investing a significant portion of available resources in system enhancements.

The high payoff derived from system enhancements provides the key to a successful strategy for the planning of systems in general: install new and replacement systems at their most basic level, but delay adding enhancements until users have become thoroughly familiar with a system and have had ample opportunity for evaluating it in operation. Such a strategy is likely to provide systems more valuable than those installed without any practical experience with the system.

Planning Systems that Enhance Management Information

Plan systems that not only process hospital transactions, but also benefit from the ability of personnel handling operational transactions to collect accurate and timely information as a by-product of those transactions. Information collected in this manner is subjected to effective, natural controls that ensure that collected data are accurate. For example, department managers are likely to report any errors in revenue record keeping simply because such errors would otherwise misrepresent their departments' performance.

Planning Systems that Provide Linkages

Systems that bridge boundaries of institutions provide important linkages. For example, systems that link the hospital, physician, and patient together will enhance patient care by providing better access to patient data, and will bond the physician more closely with the hospital and potentially increase the likelihood that the physician will admit most patients to that hospital. Systems that provide linkages with referral hospitals will provide data to improve the continuity of care and will also build strong ties with referral hospitals. Systems that link the hospital with payers may accelerate processing of claims and improve cash flow.

Systems that span typically separate business units or subsidiaries within the institution will enable the institution to eventually reap the benefits of enhanced work linkages. For example, one might consider planning to consolidate record keeping for outpatients and inpatients to standardize work processes and allow a universal registration process, performed in any one of several work locations. Not all business units, however, will value these potential linkages. Some may deliberately proceed to select incompatible technology to make future linkage more difficult to achieve, perhaps out of fear that a later change in management philosophy might make computer control more centralized, or simply to maintain autonomy in their operations.

Planning Occasional Ventures for Competitive Purposes

Some computer information systems are intrinsically valuable because they help institutions to compete, giving one institution an advantage over another. Unfortunately, such systems seldom can be purchased from a vendor. Moreover, if such a system is available from a vendor, it is available to any institution and, therefore, is unlikely to have competitive value. Furthermore, if a vendor were to be engaged to develop such a system, that system may eventually become an industry prototype from which other institutions benefit—after the original institution expended the effort and expense to develop the system.

Despite these drawbacks, a health care institution may occasionally decide to invest in information systems venture projects, both to encourage innovation and to gain a competitive advantage, at least over the short term. Carefully evaluating feasibility before approving any venture, and planning these projects just as venture managers plan their investments, will ensure that successful projects continue and unsuccessful projects are discontinued. For example, development of a pilot version of such a venture system, with further progress undertaken as a series of steps, each requiring approval before going on to the next, is likely to enable the hospital to continuously evaluate each venture project.

Planning the Enabling Technology of the Future

The usefulness of individual computer information systems is dependent on the capabilities of the underlying technological base, often called the *enabling technology* or *infrastructure,* requiring that it too be carefully planned. The enabling technology is built by selecting from among hardware and software components that are being continually improved. The greatest-capability and least-cost alternatives will be derived by carefully selecting each expansion, addition, or replacement.

Hidden costs and problems proliferate as customers' options and alternatives in selecting information technology products continue to multiply and grow more complex. Meanwhile, the complex integration of new products into existing systems remains a prerequisite for successful use of information technology. For example, a new generation of disk storage units has evolved every three or four years since the first units became available more than 20 years ago. New generations are always larger, faster, more reliable, and cheaper. And, like stock market decisions, timing is important: waiting too long to make a commitment or committing too early can both be serious mistakes. Consequently, decisions regarding technology replacement, purchasing, and leasing must be meshed well with plans for the life cycles of the hospital's systems and processes.

Planning of the enabling technology is becoming increasingly complex because evolving technology requires that layer upon dependent layer of computer hardware and software must work together to provide function. Furthermore, the underlying enabling technology is becoming highly dependent on the capabilities of data communications hardware and software. In addition, special utility software must be acquired to support functions such as the copying of data files, necessary for backup and recovery. Moreover, periodic upgrades are needed in each technical layer and within each of several technological functions, both in hardware and software, to maintain compatibility with the latest software products as they become available.

Upgrades to the underlying technology must constantly be planned and installed so that the hospital will be able to capitalize on future applications software. Flexible, high-speed interconnections among computers, for example, is an important future requirement. Another, possibly more distant, future requirement is the ability to accommodate computerized processing of integrated diagnostics: the collection and combined processing of data, text, graphics, and digitized radiology film images, for example.

Because of the complexity of current and developing information technology, special software is required for detailed utilization statistics and related performance measurement and capacity management. These and other record-keeping and tracking methods provide the performance analysis necessary to plan in today's complex information technology environment.

The Insufficiency of Traditional Planning Principles

Information systems planning principles at one time promoted painstaking study and thorough documentation of existing business procedures.[6] They prescribed extensive interviews with users and potential users of computer information systems to determine user requirements in detail. After the written products of these efforts were completed and stored in binders, feasibility studies and subsequent economic justification studies were conducted. One example of this process, known as *business systems planning,* required that entire departments' functions be completely documented in flowcharts and on special forms. In short, these principles relied heavily on the thesis that functions should be automated based either on expected cost savings or, in some cases, on possible increased profits from performing existing tasks using computer automation.

Although these endeavors are often launched with great hopes, they often encounter major problems. First, only large organizations could afford such elaborate analyses. And, during the many months required to complete such an analysis, the organizational, business, and technological environments usually change. Even if the study results are still valid at the end of the study, the results may be difficult to translate into useful support systems and could, in fact, be outdated before they are completed. Information technology inherently has a short life cycle, and more capable and less expensive newer technology may become available during the project, raising doubts about continuing the project. In addition, organizational needs change unpredictably during the life of a project: people in key jobs change, the business changes; and the organization itself may change, leading, lagging behind, or keeping pace with a changing business marketplace. The institution may undergo structural changes prompted by mergers or by the decisions of executives who fail to recognize the resulting effects on information systems capabilities and projects.

Institutions that have attempted to use the principles of the past have spent a great deal of time and money creating formal and detailed five-year plans for publication and display, only to find them out-of-date and useless within a short time. These institutions have undergone the mind-numbing process of routinely manufacturing a document instead of stimulating a sensitive focus on the institution's real opportunities.[7]

An information systems strategy or long-range plan simply does not require five-year systems schedules or detailed flowcharts describing how hospital departments function. Instead, the successful planning process senses and responds to larger forces. It focuses on the health care market and on the corporation's overall goals, strategies, and objectives. And it focuses on the enabling technological architecture and how its ongoing evolution can offer new opportunities.

In the constant flux of this environment, no static plan will suffice. Only a flexible and sensitively designed process will succeed. Examples of hospitals that have implemented a formal, cyclic, but straightforward, planning process, include larger institutions, such as The Methodist Hospital in Houston,[8] Parkland Hospital in Dallas,[9] St. Francis Regional Medical Center in Wichita, Kansas,[10] and Deaconess Hospital in St. Louis,[11] and smaller institutions, such as Children's Hospital in Columbus, Ohio.[12] The planning processes of these hospitals are similar and are designed to sense ideas and proposals at all levels of the institution, assess problems and opportunities, assess progress on current projects, revise plans in the light of new information, and allocate resources accordingly. These hospitals, and many others, have in place variations of the dynamic planning process described below.

In short, information systems planning should be conducted by both large and small health care institutions. The direction-setting influence of the planning cycle will vary across different health care institutions; its activity and effect will depend on how dynamic the institution is that it serves.

The Steering Committee: A Vehicle for Consensus and Agreement

A sound information technology plan under these challenging conditions, in both large and small hospitals, will evolve most satisfactorily in a cyclic process that is guided by a top-management steering committee, a process now in use in many hospitals.[13-16] In a large hospital, this committee includes the chief operating officer, possibly the chief executive officer, the executive responsible for information systems, and executives responsible for the hospital's major operating units (including clinical activities), and possibly one or more members of the medical staff. In a smaller hospital, the steering committee would include department managers for the information systems, finance, and other major departments, and would possibly also include one or more members of the medical staff.

As its initial activity in the first phase of planning, the steering committee assesses the institution's entire portfolio of existing information systems, identifies problems and short-term requirements, and establishes direction. This initial committee directive is an effective means of discouraging parochial attitudes of individual operating units from ignoring the computer technological plan of the institution, and it should lead to a balanced initial plan. Moreover, the initial cooperative effort of steering committee members establishes overall project priorities and initial project approvals that have the support of the entire committee. Formal periodic meetings of the steering committee monitor the progress of approved projects, reconsider priorities when appropriate, and select later projects for approval.

Developing an Annual Planning Process within a Long-Term Strategic Framework

A well-designed planning process includes several formal documents, and it also provides a means to review and reassess those documents in an organized manner.[17,18] The broadest, highest-level planning document is the combined corporate plan and information systems plan. This document includes the information systems plan for a midrange period, up to about three years, and the formal corporate plan, which provides a focus on the continually changing business environment and on a broad set of long-term strategic goals. In addition, a specific technical plan and a well-defined applications systems plan should be formulated to cover at least the first two years. Within the information systems department or division, planning is further governed by the approved current year's budget, and the following year's activities are defined by an evolving proposed annual budget. A set of specific annual goals and objectives is associated with the current year's budget, with a new set evolving for the following year.

The technical plan delineates activities for building the underlying enabling technology required to fulfill objectives set down in the broad, long-term plans. Without a specific technical plan, the institution may find itself in a web of overlapping and incompatible technology that imposes significant hidden support costs, such as the support and maintenance of several different types of networking technology. The technical plan specifically schedules technology installation activities for up to two years, and it also includes tasks that define objectives and analyze alternatives beyond two years. Typical tasks include defining new operating procedures and standards, enhancing computer processing schedules and data security, and planning for future installation of computer equipment.

The application systems plan contains three distinct groups of projects: those that have been specifically approved by the steering committee, those that have been recently completed, and those that are not yet approved. The lists, approved through several levels of review, are collectively called the applications systems plan. The plan lists all applications systems projects that are under way, recently completed, and planned. As shown in Exhibit 2.3, it includes, for each project, a project description, priority, and estimated level of effort required.

A statement of annual goals and objectives for each year is prepared during the budgeting cycle and approved late in the calendar year as the budget is being finalized. Quarterly status reports are completed throughout the year, as shown in the example in Exhibit 2.4.

Exhibit 2.3 An Example of an Application Systems Plan

Information Services Division
Applications Systems Plan
Status of Projects Completed since Last Steering Committee Meeting
As of 05/24/89

Control Number	Priority	Project Description	Department Requesting	Date Requested	Current Status	Estimated Staff-Days	Remaining Staff-Days
890017	1	Add data element to reflect employee's experience in position	Patient services	01/09/89	Complete	008	000
880148	2	New report for monthly & executive payroll due to change in FICA tax requirement	Budget control	07/01/88	Complete	020	000

Legend: 1 Immediate 2 Critical 3 Necessary 4 Highly justified 5 Less justified 6 Future 7 Pending review

Continued

Exhibit 2.3 Continued

Information Services Division
Applications Systems Plan
Status of Projects Underway
As of 05/24/89

Control Number	Priority	Project Description	Department Requesting	Date Requested	Current Status	Estimated Staff-Days	Remaining Staff-Days
880230	1	New report to track dollars for various differentials	Nursing	11/23/88	Under way	020	018
880204	1	Report to summarize employee turnover statistics	Human resources	11/01/88	Under way	007	004

Legend: 1 Immediate   2 Critical   3 Necessary   4 Highly justified   5 Less justified   6 Future   7 Pending review

Information Services Division
Applications Systems Plan
Status of Projects Requested, Not Yet Approved
As of 05/24/89

Control Number	Priority	Project Description	Department Requesting	Date Requested	Current Status	Estimated Staff-Days	Remaining Staff-Days
880236	4	Maintain beneficiary data in on-line system	Benefits	11/22/88		040	040
880246	4	Implement health clinic feature to record physician exams & dates	Human resources	09/18/88		030	030

Legend: 1 Immediate 2 Critical 3 Necessary 4 Highly justified 5 Less justified 6 Future 7 Pending review

Exhibit 2.4   An Example of a Quarterly Status Report on Annual Goals
and Objectives

Annual Goals and Objectives
First Quarter Status Report

Category/Goal	*Persons Responsible*
Promote high-quality patient care:	
• Continue to add results reporting to additional departments to allow display of patient test results for physicians and nursing personnel.	John Jane
Status: Digestive disease results reporting capability was completed. Development of social services results is under way.	
• Install pharmacy computer system for enhanced management of medication dispensing and inventory.	Mary David
Status: Contract negotiation under way.	
Enhance systems in support of operations management, including enhancements to financial and human resources systems:	
• Implement the cost-accounting system, and train users to utilize the information for broad analyses. Provide good access to an accurate data base, and provide for broad end-user computing for management reporting with adequate data controls. Also provide for an analysis of departmental productivity.	Catherine Ken
Status: The cost-accounting system has been implemented into production. Patient information has been loaded and used to analyze accuracy.	
Continue to improve management processes of the Information Services Division:	
• Automate the divisional manual. Make it on-line as well as on paper.	Betty
Status: Under way	

These documents are used throughout the annual planning cycle. Early working documents are discussed, reevaluated, modified, and forged into formal documents that also evolve continually. When this planning process is executed well, each step of the cycle generates new information that leads participants to important new conclusions or to new issues that must be addressed.[19,20] Also, as strategy and plans lead to execution and implementation, the organization evolves. These conclusions and issues, and the organization's evolution, in turn affect the next step in the cycle.

Step 1 of the Annual Cycle: Environmental Analysis

The first formal step in each annual planning cycle is an environmental analysis that focuses on a thorough reevaluation of new opportunities available through information technology. It may be structured around a one- or two-day conference that includes presentations to assembled information services managers, other hospital managers, and technical experts by selected vendors, consultants, and other experts. Vendors present emerging and future versions of their products; consultants and other experts present information about new concepts, new technology, and emerging products. These presentations, followed by question-and-answer sessions, provide an opportunity to assess significant shifts in business and technology. In a larger or more dynamic institution, or one in a state of rapid change for any reason, a similar analysis is conducted as Step 5, in the latter part of the yearly cycle. Both are designed to provide learning and data-gathering experiences unavailable in the daily work environment.

This planning step, however, is only a means to focus all the forces that may contribute to changes in the plans. As Figure 2.1 shows, the spring environmental analysis is the first of six planning steps of an annual planning cycle. The six rectangles in the horizontal row through the figure represent the six steps. In each step certain plans and issues are reviewed and analyzed, indicated by the arrows pointing into the rectangle, and certain plans are updated, indicated by the arrows pointing out of the rectangle. Formal, corporate planning documents are at the top, while divisional and other plans are at the bottom. The circles in the matrix indicate the relevance of that planning item to that step. As the figure shows, the environmental analysis also requires a review of the technical plan and the application systems plan.

Additionally, all new information technology proposals and project requests submitted by departments and project teams are consolidated and reviewed during this step. This allows bottom-up input from many of the people who will ultimately be affected by the resulting plans. Some requests come from members of information systems project teams, diverse working

Figure 2.1 Information Systems Annual Planning Cycle

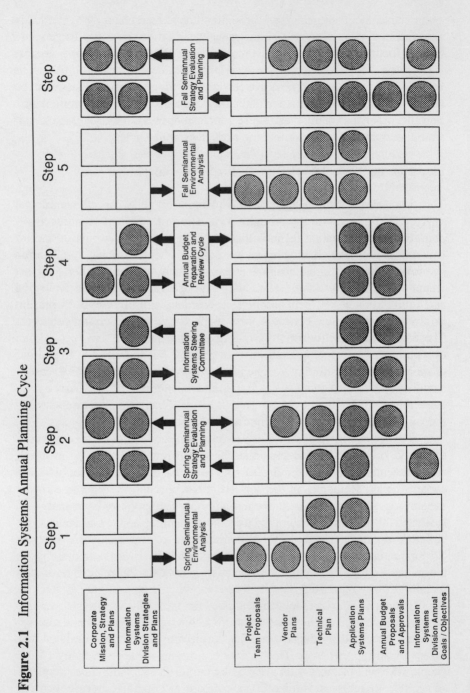

groups that are assigned to implement approved projects. Other requests come from system users, who prepare written requests that may be reviewed by project teams. Some project requests come from members of the steering committee, while still others are dictated by the corporate plan. As shown in Exhibit 2.5, project requests are recorded on forms that include a description of the request, its justification, and comments regarding timing or importance, and that allow subsequent appendage of both additional information and approval signatures. After each step in the annual planning cycle, information is channeled back to the requesters, keeping them abreast of new directions and their implications while also stimulating the identification of new opportunities.

To complete the environmental analysis, proposed additions and changes to the applications systems plan are consolidated and recorded, proposed changes to the technical plan are recorded, and items that may affect the next annual budgeting cycle, still many months away, are defined for deliberation during the budgeting cycle. Finally, specific action items are assigned in preparation for the next step in the planning cycle, the evaluation and updating of plans, which will take place four to eight weeks later. This next step consolidates all new and changed information, looks inward with scrutiny, and defines specific changes to various plans.

Step 2: Evaluation and Updating of Plans

Like the environmental analysis step, the evaluation and updating of plans step may be structured around a one- or two-day conference attended by management and staff of the information services departments. As shown in Figure 2.1, strategy evaluation requires participants to review the corporate plan, the information systems plan, the technical plan, and the application systems plan. Research and follow-up items assigned during the environmental analysis are discussed as agenda items, and progress on current year goals and objectives is examined to identify new developments and deviations. Additionally, items on the technical plan and application systems plan are updated, and specific product information may be formally requested from vendors. Once again, items are recorded for the annual budgeting cycle.

Proposed changes to the applications systems plan and major changes to the technical plan are specifically identified and prepared for discussion with the information services steering committee, since these changes may affect the budgeting cycle that is about to begin. Consensus here is vital: budget items must be understood, and they must be agreeable to, and approved by, executives of other hospital entities, which may receive smaller

Exhibit 2.5 An Example of a Project Request Form

Information Services Division
Project Request

Instructions: 1. Complete the top portion of the form.
2. Attach any necessary supporting documentation.
3. Obtain managerial approval prior to submission.
4. Submit form to the Information Services Division

Requestor: _____ Date: _____

Title: _____ Phone: _____

Division: _____ Mail station: _____

Department cc#: _____ Department name: _____

Type of Request: Date required: _____

☐ HIS screen changes   ☐ New or replacement   ☐ Staffing/work flow
☐ HIS report changes   system project   analysis
☐ Profile/table changes   ☐ Systems analysis   ☐ Statistical/graphical
☐ New report creation   ☐ Operational audit   data analysis
☐ System enhancement   ☐ Survey design/   ☐ Other: _____
                                 analysis

Project Description:

Reason for Change/Statement of Benefit:

Manager approval: _____ Date: _____
Sr. vice president approval: _____ Date: _____

ISD Project Control:

Project title: _____ Control #: _____

Date rec'd: _____ ISD dept. responsible: _____

Estimated required staff-days: _____ Elapsed time (weeks): _____

Aproved as priority: _____ by: _____ Date: _____

Other comments: _____

Final user acceptance by: _____ Date: _____

Revised 3/89

portions of available budget funds as a result of allocations to information technology projects.

Step 3: Steering Committee Review of Plans

A special meeting of the information services steering committee should follow the spring environmental analysis and strategy evaluation steps in the annual planning cycle. This committee, the highest-level executive group that reviews and approves information technology plans, includes representatives from all the hospital's major divisions and, possibly, the medical staff. Committee members generally meet quarterly to review current applications systems plan projects, set priorities, and approve projects. Their agenda is determined by summary reports prepared as part of environmental analyses and strategy evaluations.

Steering committee meetings enable top decision makers to review plans and progress and possibly to approve changes to the plans. Many different agenda formats are workable. At The Methodist Hospital in Houston, three reports are prepared for this purpose, the reports that collectively make up the applications systems plan, shown in Exhibit 2.3. One report summarizes all projects completed since the committee's last meeting, while a second report covers all projects approved and under way. The third report focuses on two types of projects: those projects previously considered and validated but not yet approved, and those projects that have been reviewed by project teams and others but not yet by the steering committee. Discussion might also center on determining which projects will be approved at the next steering committee meeting or before a significant institutional event, such as the opening of a new building. The best of both the bottom-up and top-down approaches to planning are made possible in this type of planning process.

Between steering committee meetings, procedures must be in place to accommodate high-priority projects that arise suddenly. Any project not previously planned should be sponsored and proposed by a committee member, then approved by a designated executive, such as the chief operating officer or chief executive officer, who should first discuss and agree with other committee members on priority and justification.

As major decision makers of the institution, members of the steering committee are usually also involved with the annual review of, and potential changes to, the corporate plan. Through discussions about information technology at steering committee meetings, these executives are made more aware of potential information technology opportunities that might be relevant to any corporate plan changes that are under consideration.

Step 4: Integration with the Annual Budgeting Cycle

As shown in Figure 2.1, the fourth step in the planning cycle is the annual budgeting process. In most institutions, where the fiscal year coincides with the calendar year, budgeting begins in late summer and continues through late fall. If funds are available and budget items are approved during this process, planned projects then become part of planned objectives and commitments for the following year.

Step 5: Fall Environmental Analysis

When the annual budget process is complete, a large institution, or one that is undergoing great change, may continue the planning cycle with a fall counterpart of activities that took place during the early part of the annual cycle. During this second environmental analysis, the focus again shifts outward, toward obtaining relevant information from vendors and consultants. Results of the annual budgeting process are also reviewed, and if budget expectations were not attained, redirection may be required. At this point, the end of the annual cycle is approaching and preparations for the new year begin.

Step 6: Fall Evaluation and Updating of Plans

In organizations that choose to undertake a fall counterpart of activities of Step 2, this becomes the final step in the annual planning cycle. The technical plan and applications systems plans are reviewed and updated to reflect changes necessitated by the budget cycle and other influences. In addition, the corporate plan may have changed as a result of its annual review cycle, and any changes made to it are examined and discussed. Exhibit 2.6 illustrates the linkage of the corporate plan and the information systems plan. The first column lists elements in the corporate plan, while the second and third columns describe items that form the foundation of the information systems plan. To establish goals, the second column identifies the critical information technology objective necessary to support the corresponding corporate plan items. From these, specific action tasks are defined for the information systems plan. As the corporate plan changes, the critical information technology objectives on which that corporate plan item depends are updated, reshaping the information systems plan accordingly.

Finally, goals and objectives for the next year are finalized and assigned to individuals or project teams. Publishing the list of goals and objectives in a conspicuous manner enables employees to sense how their efforts

Exhibit 2.6   An Example of Linkage of the Corporation Plan and the
Information Systems Plan

Corporate Plan to the Year 2000	*Critical Objective for Information Services Technology*	*Information Services Division Strategies and Plans of Action*
Provide mechanisms that improve the efficiency of physicians' private practices.		
• Link physician offices with hospitals through computer networks.	Computer, telecommunications, and software support to build valuable information links.	*Strategy:* Provide a range of innovative capabilities to assist physicians and their staff by providing services that we can uniquely offer, such as links for inquiry on patient results, detailed data on procedures offered at the hospital, including links from a distant physician's office. Evaluate the value to physicians of these capabilities.

Plan: Install connections first to physicians in connected campus buildings for financial and patient test results data. Link next to distant physicians on the medical staff. Offer all physicians an access code. Develop a single set of procedures for all accesses, so that new training and awkward procedures do not result. Install highly secure telecommunications hardware to protect patient data access. Add access to surgery schedule when available. Add links from distant hospitals when justified. |

relate to the goals of both the division and the hospital, and keeps them abreast of status and progress. Information systems employees can be invited to voluntarily assume responsibility for some of the work items on the list of goals and objectives, items that might otherwise fall outside their assigned scopes of responsibility. This method allows the institution to benefit from additional staff work without making permanent staff assignments. Line employees are usually enthusiastic about taking responsibility for the special effort because the experience broadens their careers.

The Result: A Relevant and Useful Planning Process

Information technology planning that is organized, clear, and relevant to corporate goals has a direct impact on an organization's ability to make directed, consistent, and effective progress. Detailed plans stipulating timing and personnel requirements reduce the risk of failure that could result from spreading personnel too thinly over projects. Clear and well-aimed information technology plans also are crucial to maintaining high-quality technological decisions. Detailed planning and reference to medium- and long-term objectives, for example, clarify issues of timing and interdependencies of technology components, and allow selection of an optimal combination of lease agreements and purchase strategies for acquisition of new equipment. Additionally, a widely distributed, well-understood plan becomes the all-important base of the next planning cycle.

As the technical plan, the application systems plan, the annual goals and objectives, and the information systems plan as an appendage to the corporate plan become a part of each hospital's culture, they become the subjects of meetings and discussions, bringing groups of people together to work toward successfully absorbing future waves of change. Consequently, the planning process is an effective means of communication, helping build awareness and understanding of new concepts. Moreover, planning affords considerable value as a means for consensus building. The planning process helps to integrate disparate views that are found within every organization. Understanding and agreement build motivation and enthusiasm that can help to bring the plan to fruition. Once people understand and identify with plans for the future, they are willing to invest effort beyond normal work levels to make them happen.

Despite a thorough planning process, a well-understood strategy, and a successful track record, the annual planning cycle is, nevertheless, vulnerable to subversion from within the organization. Ambitious users may attempt to dictate new and replacement systems favorable to their own self-interest and political motivations rather than to the welfare of the institution as a whole. Self-serving users may also attempt to subvert the planning process to weaken its credibility as an effective means of determining directions and priorities for use of information technology.

Ironically, another potential difficulty springs from the very success of this planning process. With effective planning and an established and consistent record of achievement, the temptation may arise to force certain technology beyond its capacity or functional capability. Requests may be made to modify the software "one more time," pushing it to do something that it was never planned to do, and consequently driving the hardware and software to perform additional processing that could jeopardize reliability.

A successful planning process encourages reaching beyond the simple automation of what the business currently does manually. It considers and capitalizes on the organization's long-term objectives, generating information systems enhancements that not only support them, but that also actually drive the organization toward its objectives. The process fosters a steady stream of information services innovations that enhance both the institution's operations and its products.

The planning process eliminates the tendency to develop plans based on what other hospitals are doing or to choose software packages from what vendors promote in their marketing efforts. It also neutralizes vendors' efforts to maneuver the promise of information systems into the slightest and least-important need of an unprepared client.

Because the planning necessary to select an appropriate portfolio of high-quality information systems is difficult, some executives may be tempted to sidestep, or diplomatically avoid, the problems and frictions that determined management of an orderly planning process may involve. Careful planning has become an absolute necessity, however, as unavoidable limitations on corporate budgets require the institution to face difficult choices while carefully managing the evolution of an information systems portfolio that will help ensure the hospital's success. Ultimately, the value of planning lies not merely in the plan that is produced, but in the power of a continuing process. An uncertain, dynamic health care industry and information technology marketplace invalidate any other approach.

Notes

1. F. W. McFarlan and J. L. McKenney, *Corporate Information Systems Management: The Issues Facing Senior Executives* (Homewood, IL: Richard D. Irwin, Inc., 1983), pp. 68–73.

2. B. Minard, "Managing the Hospital's Portfolio of Information Systems," *Healthcare Strategic Management* 5, no. 1 (1987): 16–22.

3. D. W. Warner, D. C. Holloway, and K. L. Grazier, *Decision Making and Control for Health Administration* (Ann Arbor, MI: Health Administration Press, 1984), pp. 6–15.

4. B. Minard, "Effective Information Systems Planning," *Computers in Healthcare* (July 1987): 40–48.

5. G. M. Murray, "Information Management: Growing Up at Children's," *Healthcare Information Management* 2, no. 3 (Fall 1988): 2–4.

6. IBM Corporation, *Business Systems Planning: Information Systems Planning Guide,* Document GE20-0527-3, 4th edition, July 1984.

7. McFarlan and McKenney, *Corporate Information Systems Management,* p. 74.

8. B. Minard, "Growth and Change Through Information Management," *Hospital & Health Services Administration* 32, no. 3 (August 1987): 307–18.

9. G. Kolenaty, "Hospital Information Systems Planning," in *Information Systems for Patient Care,* ed. B. I. Blum (New York: Springer-Verlag, 1984), pp. 147–64.

10. S. Denger, D. Cole, and H. Walker, "Implementing an Integrated Clinical Information System," *Journal of Nursing Administration* 18, no. 12 (December 1988): 28–34.

11. H. H. Schmitz, *Managing Health Care Information Resources* (Rockville, MD: Aspen Publishers, 1987), pp. 119–42.

12. G. M. Murray, "The Coordination of Corporate Strategic Planning and Information Management," presentation at ECHO (Electronic Computing Health Oriented) Conference, September 1988.

13. Minard, "Growth and Change."

14. Murray, "Information Management."

15. N. M. Lorenzi and E. B. Marks, "University of Cincinnati Medical Center: Integrating Information," *Bulletin of the Medical Library Association* 76, no. 3 (July 1988): 231–36.

16. Denger, Cole, and Walker, "Implementing an Integrated Clinical Information System."

17. Minard, "Effective Information Systems Planning."

18. Murray, "Information Management."

19. Minard, "Effective Information Systems Planning."

20. Murray, "Information Management."

3

ORGANIZATION AND MANAGEMENT

In today's dynamic health care industry, management processes and organizational structure are inextricably bound to the use of information technology. A health care institution must manage well in order to use effectively the information technology that supports its management systems. At the same time, with successful use of information technology bolstering the institution's management processes, new and useful management methods become available. In short, the creative use of information technology and creative management methods breed each other.

An Opportunity to Control and Manage Change

The need to implement new information technology and management methods provides a special opportunity for top management to create, control, and manage change. They may choose a strategy of responding to the opportunities that change naturally brings, or they may create change and then actively exploit it. Whatever the strategy, management's objective must be to develop an organizational structure and internal processes that strengthen the ability to execute and manage change. This ability to respond aggressively to change is vital to the very survival of health care institutions because the volatility of the health care business environment presents both problems and opportunities. Information technology can serve as a fundamental catalyst for incorporating change. It may be used directly to automate work processes and to function as the main component of a new or changed institutional process or a means to accomplish an important objective, such as to provide patient test results directly to physicians in their offices. Its use may also have an indirect benefit on the periphery of automated functions, where it may indirectly be used to focus scrutiny on the institution's quality of services or efficiency levels, such as in raising new questions among physicians on the responsiveness of ancillary departments in providing those patient test results.[1,2]

How an institution tolerates and assimilates change is one of its most important dimensions. Although often unacknowledged, the ability to manage change must be carefully developed, driven, and nurtured like any other asset. Information systems projects can be excellent agents for change when they are successfully guided by top management's participation and leadership, the effective work of project team participants, and carefully chosen information systems management methods.

But while organized change unleashes organizational power, it also unleashes considerable stress.[3] For example, pressing for systems and procedural changes that improve productivity, doing more and more with less and less, creates great stress in an institution, even when the change is understood to be clearly justified and feasible. Careful management of the pace of change is extremely important in preserving and maximizing the quality of an institution's work and the quality of teamwork and relationships among people working together.

Additionally, when one department is automated while an associated department is not, separate and conflicting work environments develop and artificial boundaries appear. Procedures that cross the departmental boundaries are disrupted, and the new, artificial boundaries that appear are often barriers to teamwork that previously existed. The many work dependencies among employees and departments may cause delays; erupting frustration and impatience may spark criticism and additional conflict. Surprises abound, no matter how much effort is invested in organizing and communicating planned change. These surprises sometimes necessitate abrupt changes in schedules and specifications, often require that work be redone, and frequently strain the thin thread of tolerance.

The challenge to management is to mold change so that participants perceive it as an opportunity, and not as a threat. Employees' perceptions strongly influence their reactions, attitudes, and performance, and those perceptions in turn critically affect the successful management of both automation projects and the changes that they bring.[4]

Traditional Organizational Structure and Information Management

Traditional organizational structures and processes of the past provided redundant paths of information to management because data collection and preparation processes were ambiguous and information that filtered through various management levels was only marginally reliable. Consequently, an important executive function involved selecting from among several potentially conflicting versions of the same data. However, when health care institutions are able to provide adequate information to executives, they depend less on the layers of middle management and institutional functions that acted primarily as conduits for information flow, and they are free to adopt new management methods. The accounting process, for example, grew from a historical need for a centralized process that obtained data as input and provided counts and consolidations as output. But this process, with its periodic cycle and controlled, structured access to only fully processed data, is no longer adequate to control the flow of management information. Accounting was simply a developmental stage that opened the door to a wider use of computers for information collection and presentation.

Data-processing departments of the past provided what amounted to an inadequate management support base for hospitals. Frequent information system shortcomings and data-processing failures became significant burdens that senior managers were forced to address. They first blamed the director of data processing. However, it was ultimately more relevant to examine how and by whom this person was managed.[5] In short, past failures were attributable to inadequate management at levels above the data-processing director.

One major problem, now widely acknowledged, was that data-processing directors generally worked out of the back office and were not properly guided by the management to whom they reported.[6] Computers were used initially for back-office tasks, to process the payroll and general ledger. Data-processing departments, born for those tasks, were initially managed as extensions of the payroll and accounting departments. Unfortunately, many organizations continue today to manage information systems as they did in the past, as if computers were still used primarily for accounting.

As executives face the task of transforming organizational structure, management practices, and information systems, they will find that there are no easy paths to the changed strategies and structures necessary for the future. Functions of the data-processing and accounting departments may be so intricately tied together that ties that bind the use of information systems almost exclusively to support of accounting systems may be difficult to break. Moreover, where independent islands of computer use have sprung up because management has not been sufficiently vigilant, integrating that existing automation with other computer departments and functions will be extremely difficult. In these cases, major renovation of the organizational structure, management control practices, and existing computer systems is required to produce an information system that satisfactorily serves the entire institution and furthers its long-term goals.

Management Principles Apply Regardless of Situation

Hospital management has the responsibility to ensure that all of the required computer system management functions be covered, either by the hospital or a vendor, or both. Therefore, the management principles of this chapter (and of other chapters discussing management principles) are relevant to all hospitals, regardless of whether or not the hospital owns and operates its own computer facility.

The principles throughout this chapter are management principles, and not technical methods, and apply to the management of the usage of the information system by the institution regardless of whether the computer is physically on site; they apply even if a vendor actually is responsible for operating the computer, correcting software problems, or installing future upgrades. Regardless of the vendor's participation, the hospital must be prepared to manage the usage of the system. For example, it is the responsibility of hospital management to manage the data security principles and their enforcement throughout the hospital, the methods of tracking of problems to ensure recovery, the methods of monitoring the types and frequencies of system errors, the choice of future system upgrades and enhancements, and the timing of future changes to the system.

Management's Role

The management of information technology, which was first used commercially in the mid-1950s, is in many ways still in its infancy. The most imposing challenge to management during three decades of computer use has been to impose an organizational structure and management control strategy on technology and usage patterns that are constantly and dramatically changing.

Structure and strategy that were applicable during earlier periods of limited, specialized information technology use are quite different from those required by the current era of complex and powerful interconnected systems. Computer capacities have grown rapidly, as has the number of computer terminals, personal computers, and applications for data bases. Skill requirements for information systems professionals have become increasingly rigorous in an environment where information system life cycles are short, and today's state-of-the-art systems will soon become obsolete. The pace and scope of technological change humbles those closest to it, who are overwhelmed by the constant learning required to select carefully from a maze of different technological alternatives.

Control through Structure

Structuring an information services organization that is independent of accounting functions is the primary prerequisite for assuring the success of an institutionwide information system.[7] Such an autonomous organization assures management of the ability to set goals and objectives beyond the narrow scope and short business cycles of the next payroll and accounting periods. Management of the information services organization, moreover, is an executive responsibility, and a high-level executive position must be carefully defined for this leadership task. Researchers have recommended that the position be independent of the financial function and report directly to the institution's chief operating officer or chief executive officer.[8-10] One study concludes that the probability of the information services organization's success correlates directly to the level of the responsible executive's rank, and that the chance of a positive outcome is virtually nonexistent when this executive is more than two levels below the organization's chief executive officer.[11] Institutions that have created such an independent leadership position frequently designate the executive who fills the post as the *chief information officer,* or CIO.[12] The term is used here to refer to the executive responsible for information services.

Establishing strong management control over the use of information technology, therefore, requires a change in organizational structure. The previous management position, which was merely a support function, must be expanded and integrated into a new structure in which the CIO plays a major leadership role, providing planning and management control over all of an institution's computer systems, not just those directly budgeted within CIO-managed cost centers.

To ensure that systems evolve in a direction that contributes to the institution's success, the executive selected to serve as CIO must possess not only considerable knowledge of the health care business, but also a thorough understanding of the criteria for successfully managing information systems projects. CIO candidates should have an advanced degree in business, management, computer science, or a health care-related discipline, substantial management skills, and extensive experience in managing the use of computer technology.

In addition, the CIO needs excellent speaking and writing skills and a broad perspective of the emerging role of health care in the community and in the nation. He or she must communicate well in order to serve effectively as a top-management liaison with an active voice in strategic planning processes. Such an individual must be capable of bringing information systems under control, focusing institutionwide efforts on applying competitive technology, and providing the visionary capacity and stamina necessary to manage the kind of nonstop change and growth that contribute significantly to an institution's success. The position demands a firm decision maker who can lead innovation, allocate resources, monitor projects, negotiate change, disseminate information, and handle differences and disturbances.

Like the chief financial officer, the CIO should report directly either to the chief executive officer (CEO) or to the chief operating officer (COO). A management structure in which the CIO is subordinate to the chief financial officer retains the greatest risk of repeating past failures. Such a structure usually either gives highest priority to the financial department's needs, or inappropriately empowers it to control other departments' access to information technology capability and data. Even if this management structure could function well for an institution, the potential for employees to perceive its authority as self-serving may doom it to failure.

Besides the CIO, the chief executive officer at most health care institutions has recently begun to take an active interest in developing well-managed information services. In fact, it is the CEO who usually seems to grasp best the requirements for an integrated plan and integrated systems. Others are not as motivated to focus on the full range of capability, and others usually cannot envision the contribution available from an integrated information management function.

Once the necessary organizational restructuring has taken place, the formation of an information services steering committee (as discussed in Chapter 2) is the most effective means of providing strategic planning, management control, and project priority, and of gaining hospitalwide support and involvement. This committee of top-level decision makers is both a vehicle for consensus and a source of guidance in arriving at a balanced plan. Its leadership plays a crucial part in preventing problems of parochial power struggles and loss of focus. For example, financial departments have traditionally pressed hardest to gain the greatest information technology support, and they have received that support because of their exclusive control over information systems functions. In the face of this power, other operating and clinical units predictably have pressed for separate and independent computer systems of their own. The steering committee acts to prevent this kind of monopoly of support and loss of focus.

The steering committee provides the direction necessary to assure that systems meet the broad requirements of the institution. For example, although the steering committee may initially plan and give priority to traditional administrative and financial systems, it should also direct that these systems be broad management information systems, not just accounting systems. And the steering committee and CIO are less likely than lower-level managers to be intimidated by vendors; they are also less apt to permit the ambiguity of unplanned stand-alone systems. Additionally, the steering committee and CIO are able to work effectively with physicians and physician groups on planning and decision making for clinical systems. Without this influence, the scientific mystique of clinical systems frequently permits the clinical expert or group with the scientific credentials on the subject to totally control the planning and selection activities.

Centralization and Decentralization

Each health care institution's executive management, and possibly its board of directors, faces a major decision about the extent to which information technology should be centralized or decentralized.[13] This decision must also deal with the possible inclusion of telephone technology and other functions, such as cable television networks, in the management structure controlled by the CIO and steering committee.

In choosing among alternative degrees of centralization, executives must address two interrelated issues. The first involves technology. Will information technology functions be served from one centralized computer facility, or will they be served by interconnecting several computer facilities that are distributed throughout the institution? The second issue focuses on planning and management control. Will individual computer systems serving different departments be centrally planned under the management control of the CIO and steering committee, as has been advocated in this, and the previous chapter, or can they be allowed to be independent of that control if pressure exists for that alternative?

Four resulting combinations are possible: (1) centralized management control with centralized computer processing, (2) centralized management control with distributed computer processing, (3) decentralized management control with centralized computer processing, and (4) decentralized management control with distributed computer processing. Although no one combination is suitable for all situations in all institutions—or even within a single institution—one of the four approaches is likely to dominate in any one institution, with variations and combinations periodically justified to manage special situations.

Most experts agree that distributed, decentralized computer processing should be available as an option.[14,15] If distributed computer processing is allowed, however, organizational processes must then be structured to integrate the work and data of distributed computers when appropriate. The so-called stand-alone, decentralized systems of the past should no longer be permitted; fully integrated systems are an absolute necessity to promote productivity and high-quality patient care among the interdependent work processes of the many caregivers within a health care institution.

The decision to centralize or decentralize planning and management control of information technology depends on the institution's long-range objectives. If growth and expansion are among the institution's primary long-range objectives, information technology is vital to these objectives, and centralized planning and control of information technology by management are imperative. Only centralized control of planning assures that objectives for the use of information technology are integrated with the institutional objectives.[16] Furthermore, when management control is centralized for these reasons, it is essential that organizational planning and related processes be structured to respond effectively to diverse departmental needs.

A strategy incorporating strong centralized management control requires executive management not only to support the authority and charter of the information services executive, but also to support the work performed by information services departments. If the information services function is unsupported and weak, that void will encourage splinter groups of employees with computer skills to grow in various departments. These splinter groups eventually function as permanent, independent entities, collectively consuming more corporate resources than a centralized information services organization would have required to accomplish identical tasks. Growing islands of information technology expertise also may generate political forces to perpetuate their independence from centralized control, leaving their contributions unmonitored and unmeasured by the steering committee and CIO. Once they have become well established, the task of bringing splinter computer groups back under executive management's control is extremely difficult.

Similar issues are raised by the decision to centralize information technology among a group of hospitals and other corporately linked health care institutions. The choice between alternative approaches again depends on the stage of management evolution and on other circumstances of the health care institutions involved. Generally, the most useful strategy is one that allows decentralized computer systems but exerts centralized planning and management control.

Within such a business structure of corporately linked but geographically dispersed health care institutions, three categories of potential systems should be planned and controlled differently:

1. Corporate systems, such as accounts payable systems, that serve the corporate business needs
2. Common systems, such as order entry systems, that provide the same functions to more than one institution
3. Local systems that are unique to a given institution

First, systems that are common systems must be identified. Although common systems may seem valuable for management reasons, such as economies of scale and potential standardization of data and procedures, it may be very difficult to use them successfully if the management of these business units is decentralized and the work, data flow, and information reporting cycles are not synchronized.

In any event, if a group of corporately linked health care institutions is strong, stable, and growing, as opposed to weak and disintegrating, strong corporate planning and management control set valuable standards and guide the planning, implementation, and operation of information technology for all institutions of the group. Vendors will likely urge local units to resist this corporate influence because vendors typically enjoy a large degree of control over the evolution of information technology in smaller client institutions. When these institutions are under the planning influence of a corporate group, however, vendors are much less likely to exert undue influence.

Accountability, Appraisal, and Evaluation by Top Management

Executive management must define specific performance reports and control processes that ensure effective management of the information services departments. These reports and processes must be meaningful to an executive audience including the CEO, the steering committee, and other members of top management; reports and processes used for management within the information services departments will not suffice. Not only must top executives define methods to appraise the management and performance of the information services departments, but they must also make certain that they are qualified to perform such an appraisal. Little guidance is available on how to attain this ideal, but experts do indicate its importance.[17] The crucial role of the executive appraisal process is not widely acknowledged primarily because the use of information technology as a critical resource is so new to top management. In short, they have had very little experience from which to gain the skill necessary to differentiate good performance from bad.

To exercise its responsibility for control, executive management must select, from among a wide range of processes and performance criteria, those it will monitor. The key to this challenge lies in choosing the few that will be most effective in triggering the type of behavior and performance desired of the information services departments.

One basic control process must be designed to guarantee both that the information services organization respects the project priorities established by the steering committee and that projects are being completed to hospital expectations and users' satisfaction. It must therefore identify and establish priority among projects approved by the steering committee. The information services department should produce periodic summary performance reports covering progress, status, and work remaining on all approved projects. However, estimating progress and work remaining on projects has traditionally been a difficult task for information services professionals and managers.[18] To counter this weakness, project teams may distribute their plans, work schedules, and meeting minutes to steering committee members for periodic review and appraisal. As an additional control mechanism, project completions should be signed by a manager in the appropriate user department.

Another control process involves budgeting and cost control. Chapter 2 described an annual planning cycle linked to the annual budgeting cycle. During that executive planning process, the annual budget is established based on projects and activities that the steering committee has approved for the next year. Monthly progress reports from the CIO explain any variances between budgeted expenditures and actual costs incurred.

Executives must also be actively concerned with the retention, recruiting, and career development of information services personnel. Standard employee turnover reports produced by the personnel department are helpful in assessing the number of employees leaving and their reasons for doing so. The personnel department may also obtain industry salary surveys for comparing salaries with those paid by other organizations. Although hospitals may enjoy a small advantage in their ability to recruit and retain employees who are motivated by health care's meaningful work, salaries must not be allowed to lag far behind those of other industries in the community.

Top management must additionally place high priority on establishing a control process that limits risk of major computer failure or disaster to the computer facility. To avert computer catastrophes, such as flood or fire, which could cripple an institution beyond recovery, a disaster recovery plan is essential for the information services organization. This disaster plan includes procedures for periodically copying data files and transporting the copies to a location distant from the computer facility. A comprehensive disaster plan also specifies contingency plans and procedures for using the copied files at some other facility if the primary computer facility is unavailable for an extended period of time.

Because executive management is not usually qualified to assess the quality of a highly complex and technical disaster recovery plan, an outside expert or consultant should be periodically engaged to help monitor and appraise this important management function. Risk management of asset loss through fraudulent or accidental practices should also be monitored periodically by an expert consultant. Likewise, processes for preventing inappropriate access to confidential information should regularly be evaluated by a qualified expert.

Performance reports also can be used to support another important control function: proper management of the computer utility. Computer performance reports are usually printouts optionally available automatically as by-products of system processing. For example, performance might be monitored using computerized work load reports, which describe how heavily the computer facility is loaded and how much of its capacity is being used. Similar reports or graphs on availability of the on-line system can help assess when and how frequently the computer facility is unavailable to users throughout the hospital, as shown in Figure 3.1. Also, as shown in Figures 3.2 and 3.3, reports or graphs on average response time of on-line system transactions measure how long users at terminals have to wait for computer response to commands entered. These reports, together with work load reports, help gauge how well technical capacities are being managed. The CIO should also provide executive management with reports summarizing frequencies of problems and their resolutions, information that helps determine the number of problems arising, their severity, and the time required to resolve them, as shown in the examples in Figures 3.4 and 3.5. Tabulated reports, graphic representations, and accompanying text all assist in monitoring performance.

Top management should monitor user satisfaction through periodic assessment. Survey questionnaires, for example, help pinpoint usefulness of computerized capability, appropriateness of training and other first-use preparations, perceived performance of the computer utility, and support available for response to problems and questions. For example, The Methodist Hospital in Houston uses computerized surveys that send questions and instructions directly to selected users' video terminals, thereby avoiding the risk that mailed surveys may be misplaced or forgotten. As shown in the survey example in Exhibit 3.1, users may be prompted and instructed at their video terminals to assess the computer work environment while they are actually using it.[19]

Figure 3.1   An Example of a Graph Showing Computer System
Availability

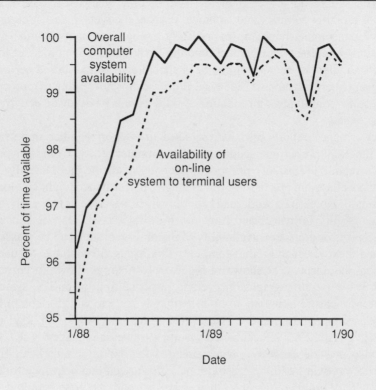

When appropriate, the CIO provides the steering committee and other top management with a written monthly report detailing progress and status and explaining cost and budget variances. This information serves as a means to review and focus early on potential problems developing in system implementation. It also provides wide communication about the status of work within the information services departments, possibly stimulating discussions of issues that may not otherwise arise. In addition, the report's clarity, accuracy, and completeness reflect the CIO's communication abilities.

Finally, top management can support its responsibility for control by requesting either periodic general audits of the information services organization or specific audits on particular topics. General audits, possibly scheduled annually as an extension of the routine financial audit, may review

Figure 3.2   An Example of a Graph Showing Average On-Line Response
Time at Video Terminals

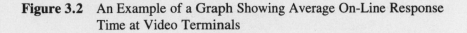

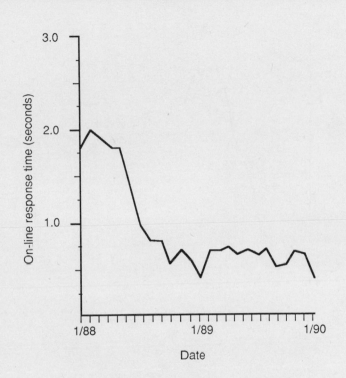

departmental procedures for appropriateness, including some checks to ensure that those procedures are being followed. Specific audits focusing on
disaster recovery procedures or data security could verify that appropriate
practices have been established and are being enforced. In addition, a special
audit may be conducted to assess how well the information services organization updates its capabilities with new versions of software and hardware.

These comprehensive practices provide vital management control. Furthermore, as they become well understood and accepted in the institution,
they trigger desirable learning and behavior in both information services
personnel and high-level executives. The chief executive officer and chief
operating officer gradually become more qualified to appraise the CIO, and
the CIO gains their confidence. Moreover, the personnel in the information

Figure 3.3   An Example of a Graph Showing On-Line Transactions with a
Response Time of Less than Five Seconds

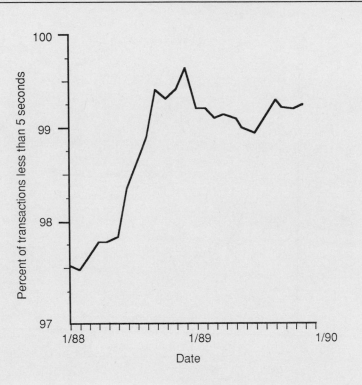

services departments come to understand and accept top management's
expectations.

Internal Management

Recent studies indicate that certain elements of internal management structure and certain skills are more important than others to the information
services organization.[20] The most crucial element of management structure
is teamwork between users and information services professionals for defining and carrying out the actual work of projects (discussed further in Chapters 6 and 7). The most important skill to the organization is the experience
and proficiency of systems analysts and programming personnel, especially
the coordinating ability and communication skills of assigned project leaders.

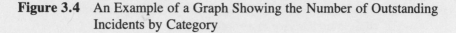

Figure 3.4 An Example of a Graph Showing the Number of Outstanding
Incidents by Category

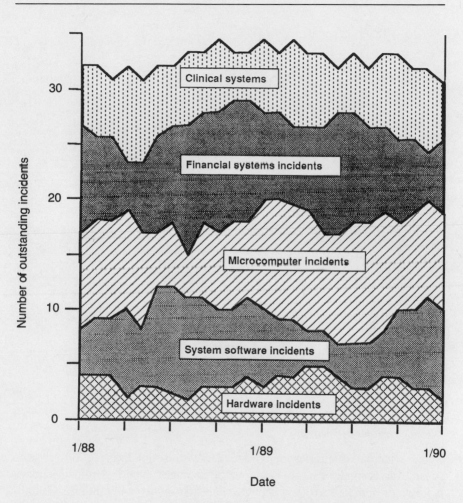

Another critical factor is the organization of work. Studies have shown that highly structured organizations with well-defined responsibilities are more likely to succeed, particularly in implementation of comprehensive integrated systems that are typical of modern health care institutions.[21] Other important factors include organizational stability, low personnel turnover, and formalized planning and project reporting.

Figure 3.5   An Example of a Graph Showing the Average Number of Days
that Incidents Are Outstanding

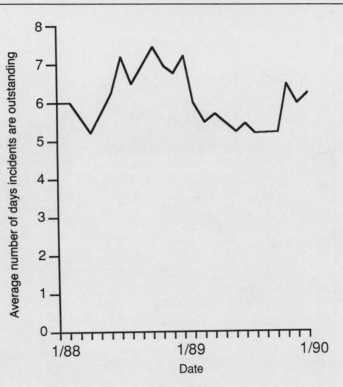

Three categories of work

Three principal categories of work exist within any information services
organization, small or large, and must be managed even if the hospital does
not own or operate its own computer. The first involves operating and managing the computer facility as a utility on which the institution depends. It
is performed by a department or function often called *computer production
services.* The second category of work, sometimes referred to as *systems
analysis and programming,* includes responsibility for implementing new
systems and enhancements to existing systems. The third category involves
planning, control, and management services, such as computer training for
users, assisting users in choosing system options, and diagnosing problems
for users throughout the hospital. An organization chart for managing the
three categories of work is shown in Figure 3.6.

Exhibit 3.1 Sample Portion of User Satisfaction Survey

We would appreciate your participation in this survey to ensure that our HIS meets our collective needs. If you do not agree to participate, select MASTER.

1. My training for physician access to the HIS was relevant.
2. Use of the HIS has enhanced my ability to provide patient care.
3. Liaison support for HIS usage is competent.
4. The second video terminal on nursing units is useful to me.
5. The system is easy to use for my purposes.

NEXT PAGE   MASTER

Computer production services. Modern health care institutions depend on information technology operations just as they do on electricity and other utilities. Information technology, therefore, should be managed as a utility is managed, maintaining continuous availability by balancing resources against needs. This task is especially difficult because conflicting and rapidly changing priorities and demands occur constantly during daily operation, with a large number of employees using the computer utility simultaneously for many different purposes. The computer utility's performance must be closely monitored, problems must be diagnosed and solved, and continuous functioning must be ensured.

The scope of computer production services covers several areas: computer operations, network operations, data entry, production control, the help desk, hardware installation and support, and technical planning and support. A sample organization chart for management of these activities is shown in Figure 3.7. In larger hospitals, these functions may be separate as they are in the figure, but in smaller hospitals, or in hospitals that use shared systems or contract for some management, the functions may be concentrated in the jobs of one or two hospital personnel.

The computer operations department actually operates the computers and processes daily work loads. Personnel of this department operate the computer using video terminal consoles, through which the system directs them to perform certain functions, such as changing paper forms in the

Figure 3.6   Information Services Organization Chart

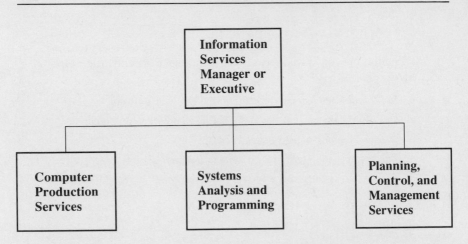

printer or loading a specific magnetic tape onto one of the tape drives. Computer operators use the same video consoles when directing the computer to perform certain functions, such as processing a particular job.

The computer operations department usually also takes responsibility for disaster recovery management, a process that involves making daily copies of important data bases or computer records that have changed and then taking those copies to a location remote from the computer center. This procedure provides vital backup in case disaster strikes the computer center, and the CIO should periodically require evidence that it works effectively. Copied data must be shown to restart processing successfully at the off-site computer center.

Computer operations personnel, or a special associated group of computer network operators, also perform a related task: operating and managing the network of computer terminals and personal computers. Malfunctions or user errors at remote computer terminals and personal computers may cause these units to cease functioning. Or a group of terminals linked to the computer through a telecommunications connection may fail because of problems in remote equipment or local telephone lines. An assigned network control operator monitors the network with support from special hardware and software that provide tools to diagnose errors, determine the number of transmission problems on telephone lines, detect symptoms of performance degradation in equipment, and restart equipment that has ceased to operate.

Data entry departments are staffed by employees with computer keyboard skills who enter data into the computer. These employees usually

Figure 3.7 Organization Chart for the Functions of Computer
Production Services

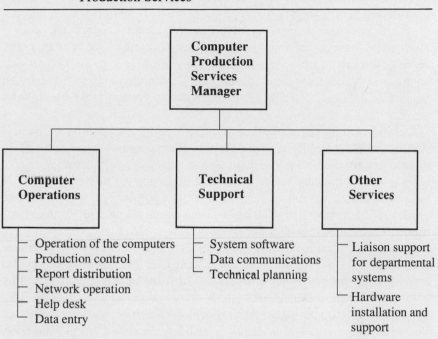

follow work schedules that the computer processing depends on, such as the entry of all patient charges before a certain time each day. During the earlier era of scheduled batch processing, data entry departments were large and crucial. Because today's on-line systems delegate much data entry to the departments generating the data, data entry departments are now dwindling in size and importance and may cease to exist within the next few years.

The department that schedules daily and other routine computer processing is known as computer scheduling or production control. This department is responsible for scheduling computer processing; ensuring that all data preparation is complete; and monitoring processing results for accuracy, the proper number of multiple copies, and outputs that conform with formats outlined in instruction documents. One way to ensure complete and accurate processing is to compare the computerized audit trail, a step-by-step listing of all tasks performed by the computer, with documented instructions. A second approach involves reviewing a computerized printout of control balances printed when a series of processing steps is completed. For example, accuracy of charge processing might be verified by reviewing sums of charges posted to all accounts, sums of revenues posted to all service departments, balance forward totals for the previous day, and balance forward totals following the posting.

The computer scheduling or production control department usually also delivers, mails, or otherwise distributes the products of computer processing—reports, checks, patient statements, and other printed forms—to appropriate offices throughout the hospital. Distribution may rely on internal mail, hand delivery, or electronic transmission to printers in the users' work areas.

Modern computer production services departments additionally include what is sometimes called a *help desk,* a telephone number users can call 24 hours a day for answers to questions and guidance in working through problems at their terminals. While some user questions are as basic as how to load paper in remote printers, help desk employees must also sometimes take immediate temporary remedial action, such as providing a replacement terminal to a user location that needs use of one immediately. Generally, the help desk staff's primary objective is to talk through and resolve problems with callers, contacting others in the information services organization for assistance and follow-up when necessary. Analysis of statistics compiled by help desk personnel can reveal both the types of problems occurring most frequently and the user departments in which problems most often develop. This information is useful in planning both system enhancements and additional user-training sessions.

The computer production services department may also have responsibility for hardware installation and support. Employees who perform this function install computer terminals and network equipment, including personal computers, and they maintain detailed records on the existence, type, and location of all equipment, computer cabling, and warranties and maintenance agreements. This group may try to diagnose problems before computer repair vendors are called, and they may even perform minor repairs. These employees also provide assistance in moving equipment necessitated by office renovations and relocations.

Finally, technical planning and technical support usually fall under the computer production services department's jurisdictions. Technical planning involves continually assessing the detailed technical performance of the institution's current information technology, analyzing the corporate and other long-term plans, and planning necessary technological evolution. Technical support is the execution of the resulting technical plan. Planning and support employees possess detailed technical knowledge of telecommunications, internal operating systems, on-line system technology, emerging computer hardware, and the complex hardware and software of local area networking.

Because personnel working in this group are highly specialized technically, they are typically more difficult to recruit.

Systems analysis and programming. Systems analysis and programming, the second major function of the information services organization, involves managing and implementing the installation of new systems and enhancement of existing systems, as shown in Figure 3.8. Various job titles define the expertise necessary to perform this work: programmer, programmer analyst, systems analyst, and project leader or project manager. The skills required for these several positions are generally similar, varying primarily in experience and job assignment. In smaller organizations, all systems analysis and programming may be organized into a single department; larger hospitals may separate support for patient and clinical systems from systems supporting traditional business processes such as payroll, personnel, and other financial functions, resulting in two separate departments each with the structure shown in Figure 3.8.

Systems analysis is typically performed by highly skilled and experienced professionals. These specialists must analyze the institutional processes proposed for automation in order to specify procedures, changed responsibilities of employees and departments, formats and contents of forms and reports, and other items that will affect or become the work of the institution's employees. These specifications are discussed and ultimately written, understood, and agreed to by representatives of hospital departments that will be affected by the new or enhanced system.

Figure 3.8   Organization Chart for Systems Analysis and Programming

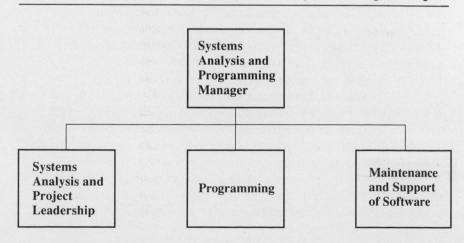

Computer programming, the next step in implementing or enhancing systems, could possibly be delegated to a more junior staff member. Programming involves writing detailed computer instructions, often in a computer language called COBOL, which has become the standard for business computer systems, or in one of several other languages typically used in clinical systems, such as MUMPS, FORTRAN, or a newer language called C. The resulting computer program is then checked as thoroughly as possible through a trial-and-error process using test data. Elimination of all potential errors is usually impossible because there are often myriad combinations of possible conditions to be tested. Errors are diagnosed and corrected in a process that continues, therefore, until management judges the value of further testing to be negligible.

After computer programming has been completed, the systems analysis skills of more experienced staff members come into play once again. They must define, organize, and manage conversions of old forms, procedures, and computer systems, as well as other preparations for use of the new system, with appropriate planning for overlap of old and new systems and procedures. Detailed instructions for usage and processing are then written, and training is subsequently conducted. These complex activities, which pave the way for the transition to the new system, involve the cooperative work of project team members, a topic that is addressed further in Chapters 6 and 7.

Project management skills play a vital role during transition activities in which critical tasks are distributed among people of several departments. Systems design and new procedures are continually reviewed at increasingly precise levels of detail, progress reviews are conducted, and judgments are made about project changes, rescheduling, or even cancellation. During the critical period following implementation, an experienced systems analyst or project manager analyzes, diagnoses, and corrects usage problems. He or she must choose from among many problem-solving alternatives in order to maintain the system in successful operational use.

For all these procedures, a skilled and competent staff is critical. The most crucial skills are those necessary to coordinate successfully the work of several people, to analyze and define systems and procedures, and to plan. Mastery of programming languages, however, especially those used in on-line systems, also is vital to the system's successful operation. Systems analysis and programming professionals also must possess the skills and instincts to build flexible, open systems for the future—systems that can easily be changed when the business environment demands it. And expertise in diagnosing and correcting problems plays an equally important role.

Planning, control, and management services. Many additional work responsibilities involve planning, control, and management services. These functions may be assigned to a separate department, added to one of the other two major work categories, or assigned to internal departmental committees including participants from both the other major work categories. The various functions that might be assigned to this separate group are shown in Figure 3.9.

Data security, one such management responsibility, could be assigned either to a planning, control, and management services group, or to the computer production services group. Data security tasks include managing access codes and passwords, ensuring that proper authority is given before assigning individual access and passwords, checking for and reviewing any questionable usage patterns, purging access codes of terminated employees, and other related monitoring. The data security function relies on automated devices such as special call-back units attached to incoming telecommunications lines, which call back incoming dial-up terminal users to verify the computerized call's origin, thereby preventing unauthorized users from accessing the system over telephone lines. Other computer system capabilities must also be in place, such as a feature that automatically signs off video terminals that are left unattended and that automatically cancels access after several unsuccessful sign-on attempts by potentially unauthorized users.

Figure 3.9 Functions of Planning, Control, and Management Services

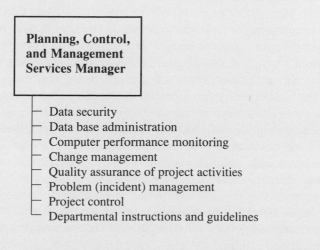

Planning, Control, and Management Services Manager

- Data security
- Data base administration
- Computer performance monitoring
- Change management
- Quality assurance of project activities
- Problem (incident) management
- Project control
- Departmental instructions and guidelines

Data security necessitates similar monitoring of access controls to data bases of confidential patient and employee data, such as those available to systems analysis and programming personnel who are implementing or maintaining systems. Data security issues are covered in greater detail in Chapter 8.

Data base administration is a similar task that could be part of the computer production services group or part of a planning, control, and management services group. This responsibility requires that an inventory of all data bases be kept, including a general cross-reference to what each is used for and what computer jobs must gain access to each. Of particular importance are data bases that are accessed through on-line systems, which must be structured and located to facilitate quick access by the computer. The data base management dilemma is much like the office management problem of determining which office files should be kept on the desk ready for immediate access, which should be kept in desk drawers for less frequent reference, and which are seldom used and should be kept in a distant file cabinet.

Special attention must be given to data bases that are accessed both by normal daily processing jobs and by on-line systems. For example, because data are added to patient accounting data bases in large batches during daily processing of patient charges, this data base must be organized serially in order to allow the efficient location of patient accounts to which charges are to be posted. In contrast, on-line processing requires that data in any patient account be quickly located in response to random inquiries by users at video terminals, who may be accessing the data base in response to telephone calls from patients requesting details of patient statements. Potential simultaneous use requires that special controls be imposed to ensure that the interdependency of these two types of access does not cause inaccuracies or usage conflicts. Here again, an office analogy may be helpful. Visualize the difficulty of managing the activity of several employees who must all use a critical office file. Without careful organization, the employees may spend their time standing in line to use the file, thereby delaying work and also delaying access to other files in the same file drawer or file cabinet.

The responsibility for computer performance management could also be delegated either to computer production services or to planning, control, and management services. This function focuses on computer capacity constraints and computer equipment limitations, using special diagnostic and measurement tools to monitor such items as response time at computer terminals, and then fine-tuning hardware and software to deliver the best possible performance. As is the case with the technical planning and technical support functions of the computer production services group, employees involved in performance management activities require skills in telecommunications, operating systems, on-line systems, computer hardware, and networking. Substantial benefits result when this function is managed well, such as gaining greater productivity, meeting more scheduled deadlines, and postponing replacement by prolonging the useful life of equipment. This does not mean that the information services organization, however well managed, can operate successfully without sufficient computer capacity, however; without adequate resources, it will certainly fail.[22]

Change management is the process by which professional programmers and technical staff employees submit a change request document to declare software or hardware changes ready for installation, and it too may be provided by either computer production services or planning, control, and management services. This process usually requires use of a special control worksheet as shown in Exhibit 3.2. It includes a description of the software or hardware change and the potential risk it poses to operations, such as the processing or users' work it may affect. Approvals are obtained from various levels of management, depending on the risks involved, with high-risk changes approved by the CIO. Whenever a change will significantly affect many users, procedures should automatically define it as high risk, thereby requiring the attention of high-level management in the information services departments. Readiness for the change and accompanying risks are analyzed by the CIO or manager who approves implementation, who may, for example, evaluate the amount of testing that was conducted. The change is then scheduled for a given date and time, depending on the affected processing cycle. A change affecting the daily cycle, for instance, may be inserted at midnight. Record keeping should include the change request document, the documented schedule of the changes (as shown in Exhibit 3.3), computerized reports of changes made to the libraries of computer programs, and follow-up tabulations of the success of the changes.

Problem management is another function that could be handled by computer production services or by a planning, control, and management services group. This responsibility involves recording the details of every reported problem, the priority of its resolution, the personnel assigned, and the continuous details of diagnosis and correction—even when it is determined to be only a simple misunderstanding. As in the sample incident report shown in Exhibit 3.4, special codes that are frequently used to categorize different types of problems provide valuable data for learning and trend reporting, planning system enhancements, and planning additional training.

Another planning, control, and management services issue involves project control. This function ensures that only approved projects are started and that projects are selected according to work priorities previously established by the steering committee. Information services personnel must not be allowed to select projects that they prefer, that are easier, or that are

Exhibit 3.2   An Example of a Change Management Worksheet

Change Management Worksheet

Risk level: Low   Emergency: Yes _____   No X

Description of change: Census report enhancements

Submitted by: Jane Doe   Phone: 2424

Submission date/time: 12/1/89   Effective date/time: 12/9/89   24:00

Change no: 18713   Related incident no: None

Special instructions: New reports, to replace existing reports

Program ID	From Library	To Library
CEN100	TEST8	PROD1
CEN120	TEST8	PROD1
CEN130	TEST8	PROD1

New documentation required? Yes _____   No X

Update required to disaster recovery plan? Yes _____   No X

Change required to reports manual? Yes X   No _____

Other change required to reports distribution? Yes _____   No X

Approved by: First level: John Smith

Second level (if required): _____

---

self-serving in any way. Periodic steering committee reports of project status provide one priority control mechanism; another develops from close work with project teams. Project team members exert a "natural" control mechanism that is extremely reliable because it is driven by the natural forces of recipients examining results and immediately reporting inaccuracies or inconsistencies, much as employees can be depended on to report errors in their paychecks.

Exhibit 3.3   An Example of a Schedule of Pending Changes

Change Management:
Report of Pending Changes

Date	Time	Change No.	Risk Level	Risk Type	Description
12/09/89	24:00	18844	Med	EMER	Correct billing problem
12/09/89	24:00	18713	Low	Norm	Census report enhancements
12/10/89	08:00	17747	Med	Norm	Updates to charge manual
12/22/89	08:00	18820	Med	Norm	New tax rates for 1990
12/31/89	24:00	17101	Med	Norm	New rates in charge manual
01/06/90	18:00	18811	High	Norm	Upgrade computer hardware

Another planning, control, and management services issue concerns quality assurance of design and programming. One useful control mechanism involves conducting a design walk-through in which assigned project team participants, both users and information services personnel, make brief presentations to assembled project team members or to a selected group of management representatives. This audience then asks questions, makes suggestions, and generally provides an audit of work in progress.

Planning, control, and management services also is responsible for preparing and maintaining an instruction manual documenting a wide range of technical and administrative standards and procedures for the information services department, including standards for naming computer programs and data bases, procedures for activities such as change management, personnel practices, and standards for data confidentiality. The manual also describes proper handling of project requests, emphasizing that priorities are set by the steering committee. For example, internal procedures might specify the methods that are to be used by users or project team members to request projects, by programmers and analysts to analyze and estimate work required, and by management and executives to approve projects.

The instruction manual also sets guidelines for project priorities and preemptions, procedures for internal management reporting, and requirements for detailed project plans and meeting minutes. Personnel administration and position descriptions also are included to ensure that personnel practices are consistently applied by supervisors throughout the entire information services organization. Recruiting practices, such as interviewing stan-

Exhibit 3.4   Sample Incident Report for Reporting Problems and
Other Incidents

Incident no: **89426**   Incident date: **12/5/89**   Incident time: **9:00**

Reported by: **Cathy Brown**

Reported to: **Alice Smith**

Dept. reported: **Nurse unit 4SW**

Assigned to: **Randy Jones**

User notifed: **Head Nurse**

Priority: **2**   Group assigned: **P**   Status: **O**   Resolved date/time:

Description: **Patient classification did not allow change to acuity**

data field.

Problem impact: **Unable to properly classify patient.**

Action taken:
Date / time		Action/status
12/5/89	9:15	Used system override to force data entry
12/5/89	15:00	Diagnosed problem, planning correction

dards and candidate selection criteria, should be covered as well. Although
definition and acceptance of standard procedures come gradually with the
organization's maturity, some standards, such as those concerning data confidentiality, should immediately be defined in order to signal the topic's
critical nature. These standards may then slowly evolve to become more
formal as specific needs arise.

Some planning, control, and management services functions are most
effectively provided through internal committees, especially if they involve

interdependencies among functions of both computer production services and systems analysis and programming. For example, change management and problem management include activities that may be handled cooperatively through committees, with one manager —possibly the manager of computer production services—responsible for the function regardless of which internal department ultimately performs the activity. A standing committee for change management might include managers from technical planning and support, computer operations, and from systems analysis and programming. Meeting weekly, this committee could review proposed changes, schedule those changes, critically review all changes that failed to work properly when installed, and take follow-up action to prevent recurrence of failure. A problem management committee composed of similar management personnel could also review, track, and analyze problems by type and frequency, subsequently proposing action, such as improved processing controls and user training, to reduce the frequency of problems or to prevent them altogether.

A similar internal committee of managers may work together with the technical planning and support group to guide technical planning. Another committee of managers and computer professionals may together guide the evolution of the computer-human interface, planning improvements in developing easier-to-use, standardized systems for users at video terminals.

Staffing management and work assignments

Productivity, as much as any other organizational characteristic, determines the information service departments' contribution to the parent health care institution's success. Productivity, in turn, is determined to a large degree by the management of staffing and work assignments within the information services departments. Staffing and work management methods, long misunderstood, traditionally have not been considered important enough to require specific guidelines originating from executive management. Consequently, they have usually been left to the routine management practices of the information services organization, with some influence from general guidelines issued by personnel departments.[23] Management issues involving staffing, assignments, recruiting, and career development are, however, extremely important. They must be defined by top management and governed by specific guidelines.[24]

Span of control

Span of control is used in organization and management theory to define the number of people that can be managed effectively by a given manager. The appropriate span of control for supervisory and management personnel hinges on the activity they supervise or manage. In the information services organization, span of control is crucial and should, therefore, be carefully determined. When an institution or its information services professionals are in a period of extensive learning and growth, span of control should be low, with no more than three or four employees reporting to each supervisor or manager. In this situation, supervisory or management personnel must devote a great deal of time to their own learning, in addition to teaching and guiding others. Likewise, if the information services organization is changing and growing, a low span of control affords supervisory and management personnel ample time to work with employees, carefully leading them through the transition. Under more routine operating conditions, span of control may be as high as seven or eight employees to each supervisor or manager.

Recruiting, retention, and career development

Recruiting, retention, and career development of information services managers and professionals requires considerable management attention. The skills of personnel assigned to project management, for example, are vital. Employees who may lead projects should be carefully recruited and selected. Managers should also be carefully chosen because they generally bear responsibility for personnel recruiting, staffing, and work assignments.

Health care institutions facing competition from local businesses and industries offering especially attractive compensation packages and other employment incentives may have difficulty recruiting and retaining information services managers and professionals. One advantage health care institutions do have, however, is the obvious and immediate meaningfulness of their work, a quality that appeals to candidates with humanitarian instincts. Ironically, health care institutions also have another competitive edge: they use information technology that is usually more modern than that used in other businesses. Industries that began using information technology much earlier have accumulated a broad base of older systems and only a narrow base of modern on-line systems. To profit from these advantages, managers should emphasize opportunities for acquiring relevant training and challenging assignments using modern technology in recruiting employees, and concentrate on maintaining a well-balanced mix of employee assignments in retaining them.

Work assignments in systems analysis and programming

The work of systems analysis and programming groups is critical to the smooth operation of the institution and must be apportioned carefully between maintenance, enhancement, and implementation of new or replacement systems. Consequently, managers and supervisors delegating assignments must consider carefully the skill level and commitment of employees under consideration for a particular task. System maintenance, for example, requires that skilled staff be assigned to current systems to keep them operating at all times. These systems must be maintained when problems occur in the programs or when recovery from a catastrophic mistake depends on the skill and dedication of the systems analyst or programmer who restores and reruns the process. At the same time, a competent manager or supervisor will always keep in mind the institution's long-term goals and assign a certain number of talented staff to new or replacement systems and enhancements to current systems, even though the functions of these systems may not yet be as critical to the operation of the institution as those long established. Competent management will also recognize that an institutional rhythm develops as a result of fluctuating emphasis on maintenance and on growth and development. Accordingly, systems analysis and programming work assignments will need to reflect that institutional rhythm.

The CIO and other members of top management are responsible for establishing guidelines for the division of systems analysis and programming staff among maintenance, enhancement, and implementation of new or replacement systems. They must also formulate broad guidelines for deciding when to replace a system that requires an inordinate amount of maintenance.

To make such critical decisions about work assignments, even in an information services organization with only a few systems analysis and programming employees, computerized record keeping can provide information helpful in pinpointing systems that require the most maintenance and those that should be selected for future enhancements or replacement. Systems analysts and programmers should routinely record the time spent on maintaining systems, enhancing systems, or implementing new or replacement systems.[25] This record keeping, the details of which could be entered through an on-line computer system as shown in Exhibit 3.5, keeps track of the effort spent on each type of activity: problem solving, making programming corrections, testing those corrections, rerunning computer processes, and other necessary activities.

Exhibit 3.6 is an example of a summary report of maintenance effort expended on a single system over a period of time, and Exhibit 3.7 is an example of a summary report of enhancements and new development effort expended on a single information systems project over a period of time. The accumulated time spent on each approved project provides data for analysis of the effort invested in system maintenance, enhancement, and installation of new or replacement systems. Summarized over all systems and projects,

Exhibit 3.5   Sample Weekly Reporting of Work Activity and Hours

Work activity for week ending: **12/15/89**

Employee: **Jane Doe**

Project: **HIS order entry system**

Project No: **890116**

Enter work hours by category:

Project meetings:
Supervision:
Other administrative:
User interview/consultation:
Analysis/design:
Programming:
Testing:
Documentation/instructions:
Training:
Implementation follow-up:
Problem diagnosis/correction:
Installing systems:
User assistance:

and displayed in graphic form, this information shows how balance among the three different activities shifts over time and also helps focus on planning and other issues involved in managing systems analysis and programming work. Figure 3.10, for example, illustrates how professional programmers spent their time during a seven-year period at The Methodist Hospital in Houston. The three separate layers represent time dedicated to maintenance, enhancement, and work on new and replacement systems.

During 1982 and 1983, staff members at this hospital devoted a fairly high level of effort to maintaining a small number of marginally functional systems. In 1984, improved management caused maintenance levels to fall steadily from May through November, while time invested in new development began to grow. By the end of 1984, approximately 80 percent of computer professionals' total available time was invested in new development, driving for the installation of a broad base of new and replacement systems late that year.

Work patterns shifted dramatically after, and because of, that milestone, with both maintenance and enhancement activity growing sharply

Exhibit 3.6   Sample Report of Maintenance Effort Expended on a System

System: Accounts Payable System

Activity	Hours This Week	Hours Year-to-Date
Project meetings	0.0	2.0
Supervision	0.0	2.0
Other administrative	0.0	1.0
User interview/consultation	1.0	17.5
Analysis/design	0.0	10.5
Programming	0.0	23.0
Testing	2.0	29.0
Documentation/instructions	0.0	12.5
Training	0.0	0.0
Installing system	0.0	8.0
Problem diagnosis/correction	2.0	16.0
User assistance	0.0	11.5
Implementation follow-up	0.0	8.0
	5.0	141.0

from November 1984 into early 1985. At the same time, new development activity was displaced, although some continuing effort was invested in developing and implementing additional computerized functions of the same broad project. The shift to increased maintenance effort was designed to support the broad new system functions installed in November 1984. Management emphasized enhancement efforts, instead of using available resources to prepare and implement additional functions, because as users became familiar with the new functions, they began defining and requesting minor changes. The decision was made, therefore, to fine-tune existing functions at the expense of accelerating installation of the remaining portions of the new system.

Maintenance levels continued to rise through February 1985, as installed enhancements generated additional system maintenance work. By April, a falling maintenance level freed some employees for work on new development, while enhancement efforts continued to grow. Maintenance work increased again in April and May, caused by the installation and start-up of major new and enhanced functions. This saw-toothed pattern continued upward through 1985, as waves of continued new functions and enhance-

Exhibit 3.7   Sample Report of Enhancement and New Development Effort
Expended on a System

Project: Cost Accounting, Integrated Patient Data Base

Activity	*Hours This Week*	*Hours Project-to-Date*
Project meetings	4.0	132.0
Supervision	0.0	18.0
Other administrative	0.0	7.0
User interviews/consultations	2.0	181.5
Analysis/design	4.5	459.0
Programming	15.0	613.0
Testing	26.0	523.0
Documentation/instruction	3.0	156.5
Training	0.0	84.0
Installing system	0.0	352.5
Problem diagnosis/correction	6.5	306.0
User assistance	8.0	62.5
Implementation follow-up	1.0	219.5
	70.0	3,114.5

ments were completed. Maintenance was then reduced to a much lower level, where it was held through mid-1986. Reduced pressure for fast-paced change permitted more attention to testing, which played a pivotal role in reducing maintenance levels. Although management approved an additional group of new and replacement systems for installation in 1986, a strong investment in system enhancements continued until mid-1986. These enhancements were controlled, however, so that during early 1986 approximately half the staff could dedicate their energies to new and replacement systems.

From a broad perspective, Figure 3.10 testifies to the long-term effects that management decisions have on staffing and work assignments.[26] During 1985, and again during 1987, the saw-toothed pattern of maintenance work had an underlying upward thrust because the steadily growing level of systems complexity and breadth created a more extensive base of systems requiring maintenance work. Although the graph illustrates monthly activity, most of the changes in slope spanned a time cycle of several months before reversing, signaling the broad strength of each effect, the power of the cause-and-effect dynamics involved, and ultimately, the importance of management decisions.

Figure 3.10 Percentage of Programmers' Time at The Methodist Hospital Spent on Maintenance, Enhancement, and New Development

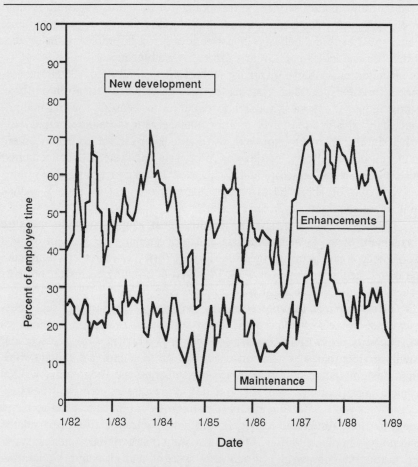

After a year of steady increase in maintenance effort, near the end of 1985 and again near the end of 1987, a downward trend occurred. Once again, employees relieved of maintenance work were assigned to new development and enhancement projects; when installed, these projects in turn led to increased maintenance requirements. At the same time, the downward trend of maintenance work signals maturity and stability in the underlying base. The reduced maintenance load allows new development projects to come to completion and then to generate yet another wave of increased maintenance.

Ideally, maintenance effort should be kept at low levels. In practice, however, management cannot afford to eliminate the need for maintenance.

Performing excessive testing in order to prevent all system errors before implementation, for example, would prolong implementation to such an extent that information services personnel and involved users would seldom complete projects. The trade-off must therefore be managed, and a suitable balance must be found between investment of effort in preparing the system for first use and investment of later effort for maintenance.

In addition to these summary statistics, detailed analysis of maintenance efforts for individual systems focuses management attention on those systems requiring the most maintenance and on the reasons for that maintenance. This clearer focus may prompt management to change employees' work assignments, make improved staffing decisions in future enhancement and development efforts, or develop proposals for system enhancements. Those proposals, subjected to additional evaluations concerning all systems involved, may be approved as enhancement efforts that eventually reduce maintenance requirements in later periods.

The same data, presented in another form, can be used to measure management of the systems analysis and programming department against that of other organizations. Figure 3.11 shows how computer professionals' time is invested in the types of work involved in bringing computer projects to successful use.[27] The most recognizable type of work, "programming," is the effort required to write computer programs. "Definition" represents systems analysis efforts required to collect a project's or system's objectives and requirements, write a request for proposal when new or replacement systems are required, and gain consensus and agreement on a detailed definition. "Design" includes systems analysis decisions and judgments, written technical specifications, and file and data transmission design. "Testing" encompasses both collection and preparation of data that are used to test a system and the systematic testing of the new programs, files, and related technology. "Implementation" involves writing instructional material, training, thoroughly comparing old and new systems and procedures operating in parallel, and other preparation for first use of systems until they are accepted by assigned project teams. "Administrative" is time spent on the work required to prepare and update project plans, attend project meetings, write meeting minutes, and perform other related supervisory duties.

The curve connecting the ends of the bars in Figure 3.11 would be roughly bell-shaped in many organizations, with programming consuming the largest chunk of available resources. As the chart illustrates, however, that was not the pattern at The Methodist Hospital in 1989. The following analysis will show the reasons for this difference; a similar examination would be useful to management in reviewing staffing and management practices in information services functions in other organizations.

Figure 3.11 Time Reported by Category for Enhancement and New Development at The Methodist Hospital in 1989

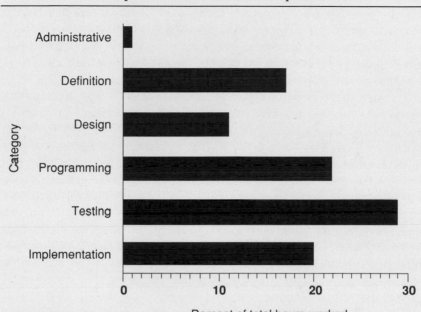

In Figure 3.11, testing effort is greater than programming effort for several reasons. Programming is lower than it might otherwise be simply because the institution's policy is to purchase or license software packages whenever possible. For this same reason, design effort is also lower. The work of system definition, on the other hand, is affected minimally by the policy of acquiring outside software packages. Because few vendor proposals meet all the needs of a large and complex hospital, a great deal of systems analysis time is required first to define modifications and extensions of the vendor proposal and then to modify existing procedures so they will match the selected system's functions.

This institution invests a modest amount of programming effort. Some programming is required to make modifications and extensions, but a great deal of programming work is also required to develop the maze of system interfaces necessary to integrate new automation with established systems and procedures. Interfaces among software packages and existing systems are usually more complex than the mainstream software on which implementation efforts are focused.

Interfaces, unique and not part of market-defined software packages, are subjected to intense testing. Special testing of these interfaces is also mandated by the large volume of transactions involved and the complexity of accommodating many necessary exceptions. Testing effort here reduces the risk of operational failures as well. Successful operation is heavily dependent on interfaces that are forced to operate in very tight time frames, typically between major information cycles of the institution, at the ends of days, or before the next cycle can successfully begin.

Therefore, as shown in Figure 3.11, testing effort is high in this institution because the systems are complex and must be tested under a great variety of conditions. The fact that software is operating in one hospital does not necessarily mean it will operate successfully in another large hospital. Testing effort is also high because one of management's guiding principles is to minimize risk by investing resources before first use of the system in order to avoid a potentially greater use of those same or equivalent resources later for problem solving. Information services employees usually accept this emphasis on testing, as do new users of automation, who have no old patterns to overcome. Most difficult to convince are small groups of users who prefer traditional methods and who don't care to devote effort and time to preventing problems, preferring instead to deal with them after system installation as they did in the past.

Work effort invested in implementation provides the same high leverage effect on system quality that testing does, and it is similarly justified.

Use of Project Teams as an Institutional Strategy

The systems analysis and programming staff performs most of its work through project teams and their related work groups of users in other hospital departments, including department managers, and including clinical personnel in cases where the project involves clinical systems. Hospitals that use project teams to define, select, and implement hospitalwide projects report that project teams create a sense of commitment and ownership,[28] generate positive attitudes and cooperation,[29] and are an invaluable source of innovative ideas, teamwork, and synergy, which do much to improve the quality of projects.[30,31]

Health care institutions that have used project teams successfully report that physicians and nurses should be well represented in project teams that are defining, selecting, and implementing clinical information systems.[32-34] As hospitals face opportunities to use advanced information systems to reduce costs and improve quality of care, decisions about clinical information systems become strategic decisions in which physicians and other clinical personnel should play a major role, since these people are especially familiar with the work processes and their problems[35] and won't tolerate definition or selection of a system that results in a productivity or quality deficiency.[36]

Physicians and nurses have typically not been well served by information technology in the past, and in some cases have been victims of others' decisions. Earlier systems were oversold, as they were expected to eliminate paper and reduce work loads, when in fact the new systems increased work loads by requiring that information be entered on forms and entered into the computer, causing the clinical personnel to perform the added work of dealing with both sets of media and methods—and they received no benefits in return. The clinical systems of the future will offer great opportunities, and will bring great change, but they will only be successful if the specific requirements and decisions of clinical personnel are carefully obtained throughout the duration of the project.

Managing Project Teams

Management methods and procedures that cross departmental boundaries, directing the collective and cooperative work of project team participants, are becoming as vital to the success of the information services organization as are its internal processes.[37] One of the CIO's most critical objectives is to ensure that the joint efforts of people working together on project teams are well managed.

In the past, information systems were defined or selected based on one department's specifications at the expense of others, imposing the requirements of the new system across that department's boundaries and onto the work processes of departments with which it shares work. In the best of cases, the result was disappointment and lost opportunities to improve interdepartmental processes.[38] In the worst of cases, the decisions crippled broad institutional processes, causing crises for the institutions involved.[39]

Project teams require close management and negotiation to unify the work of the group in defining systems that integrate the work of several departments.[40] Several health care institutions report that management must carefully negotiate issues and manage the change that occurs at departmental or political boundaries.[41–43]

Project team participants should initially be assigned to define in detail how systems must function to meet both current and future needs. A project team might be established, for example, to implement a new or replacement hospitalwide financial reporting process, an employee-based record-keeping system, or a clinical system. Assigning project team participants from all departments with a vested interest in the project's outcome, rather than exclusively from the primary department involved, ensures that all affected departments contribute to the effort, and that all would suffer from the consequences of poor-quality work. Members of the project team bear responsibility for defining and agreeing to system functions. When a product is chosen, the project team should expand to include a vendor representative. In this case, management controls must prevent vendors from attempting to force-fit their system, which may only marginally meet the hospital's requirements, undetected by other project team members.

The task of project team management requires assessing participants' competence and assigning activities based on their ability and readiness. It means fostering innovation, gaining consensus, and encouraging high productivity by team members, while also building trust and striving for high quality. The CIO demonstrates strong leadership primarily by selecting competent project team managers and work group leaders from among the information services and user management ranks, and then helping them apply team management methods. In fact, the CIO must at times serve as project manager on teams assigned to the most important projects. This process gives appropriate leadership to important projects and also establishes a model for others to follow.

Each project team manager must ensure that team members take their responsibilities seriously and do not regard the team as just another committee appointment. Emphasizing the effects of recent information systems project failures at other local institutions often helps focus attention on the gravity of the issues involved.

To manage project teams well, project managers must stimulate innovative thinking and discussions that create differing proposals, while at the same time leading the participants toward agreement. As meeting chairman, for example, the project team manager must engage silent participants, occasionally add acknowledged experts to meeting agendas, and force discussion of controversial and differing proposals. Within some project teams, creativity and consensus grow naturally from the enthusiastic participation of appropriately assigned team members. In other cases, they require stimulation from the project team manager. Once the innovative process gains momentum, it must be molded, balancing and shaping the brainstorming to meet both project and hospital needs. Important and useful innovation will likely come from employees in the organization's trenches, where actions are triggered by the work environment and by the expectations of personnel who work in closely interrelated jobs. The challenge of project team management, therefore, lies in fostering innovation by finding ways to connect these employees and help them communicate.

Each manager of a newly assigned project team must help the project team members reach a better understanding of both the information system that is to be defined and the institutional management processes that are involved or may be affected. Agendas might include a tutorial on cost accounting or clinical instrumentation, or a review of third-party reimbursement practices. Project team members must also be informed about evolving information technology capabilities and about the vendor marketplace.

Special Concerns for Complex Clinical Systems Projects

Clinical systems projects have been especially disappointing in the past. Clinical computer systems have been difficult to use and extremely costly, required long periods to implement, and added little value beyond what was possible using manual procedures.

One reason may be that medicine is very complex and is purposefully fragmented into many specialties, better suited to understanding and handling a subset of medical responsibilities.[44] Each specialty is itself very complex and its practice is stressful and difficult. Consequently, some think that physicians should participate in clinical systems projects so that the procedural changes in the work of each individual physician are kept at a minimum.[45]

Consequently, information systems projects that attempt to integrate and generalize the work processes of the many specialities of medicine and nursing are burdened by complexity and difficulty that are far beyond that of other, more conventional systems projects. The project teams must define information and automation processes that will be new and extremely complex. The system will have broad impact, affecting the daily work of hundreds, perhaps thousands, of employees and physicians. Each individual clinician understands his or her own practices and processes, but the complex interactions among the many are not well defined, and few, if any, can understand how any given system will ultimately affect the integrated work of the many.

The solution is to expend the effort necessary to define the system in terms of all the subprocesses.[46] The subprocesses are then mapped together in diagrams, associating work processes in "colonies" of work, so that each subprocess is as independent of the others as possible and functions as autonomously as possible.

Project team participants may express intolerance of the degree of detail and complexity that these tasks require. Despite prior experience and adequate training, their self-confidence may erode as they struggle with complex details of systems and procedures.[47] Faced with this intolerance, the project team manager may be tempted to defer to outside consultants to provide detailed specifications. Common in many institutions, deferring these tasks to consultants may seem to be a suitable solution and a welcome relief to project team participants; however, it deprives the institution of opportunities for innovation that would very likely flow from the detailed work of involved project team members working together on issues affecting the hospital's future capabilities. The project team manager must therefore convince team members of the need for complete definition and thorough detail, persuading them that the investment of time and effort will pay off in a more useful and successful system.

Researchers supporting this project team, or participative, method of system definition and implementation propose that in addition to its value in support of the project, this process triggers important organizational learning. Managed well, it induces managers and other project team participants to learn about each others' responsibilities and problems, systematically leading the institution to the orderly change and growth that may pave the way to a successful future.[48]

Change Management: An Emerging Management Issue

Planning and managing well in the present requires that health care executives also look constantly to the future. Such foresight is especially necessary when designing and implementing computer information systems, where today's decisions result in tomorrow's opportunities or obstacles.

New and evolving information systems possess the potential to act as catalysts for the integration of functions previously performed by independent departments. This prospective integrative role holds far-reaching implications for management.[49] As new systems are implemented, for example, newly created issues necessitate closer coordination among department managers and their staffs. Department managers and staffs are required, sometimes reluctantly, to learn about a wide range of health care issues and to understand the workings of other departments, such as room and bed management and order handling among nursing and ancillary departments. This collective learning strengthens institutions whose personnel were not pressed for such formal coordinating and integrating activity in the past.

As preparations progress for installing a new computer system, team members discuss project details and rumors begin to spread. Executive management will wisely take advantage of this opportunity to control the messages that are being disseminated and eliminate speculation and uncertainty. As a new system begins to emerge, for example, it gradually becomes apparent to the personnel of the institution that existing tasks and responsibilities will change and certain new ones will be created. Instead of simply allowing new tasks and responsibilities to emerge formlessly out of the combined work of the project team, however, management can define those new tasks and responsibilities so that the system emerges with specific procedures, controls, and changed organizational responsibilities.[50] By thus taking the initiative in defining new organizational roles and responsibilities, management also ensures an accompanying message of confidence and competence. If, on the other hand, management ignores this opportunity to control the emergence of change, institutional forces will emerge from the resulting vacuum, driven by pressures to preserve or gain power, hide information, or create new needs for experts in certain departments. New systems always create new information and new processes, and uncontrolled growth can result in the creation of jobs where they are not necessarily best for the institution. The resulting message of laissez-faire management is as damaging to institutional morale as laissez-faire growth is to performance.

Preparation for a new information system inevitably precipitates a need to focus intensely on the quality of the institution's work. During this period, with its attendant need for improving productivity, employees readily accept analysis and scrutiny of existing procedures that might otherwise be perceived as threatening.[51] The task of selectively retraining groups of employees is also more easily and diplomatically accomplished at this time. Preparing for a new system causes employees to examine and analyze their jobs and procedures, and it leads them to learn and improve more than might otherwise be possible.

When looking toward the future, it is important to remember that new information brings new power—and control of information brings a greater span of control to an institution's higher management levels.[52] Successfully prescribing systems to achieve greater use of this information power enables top management to better control FTEs (full-time equivalent positions), wages, and other costs. Where power shifts are desired, moreover, top management must make certain that prescribed systems and procedures lead to power shifts that best serve the institution. To prevent such shifts, systems and procedures must likewise be structured appropriately.

In fact, a new computer system can be the agent for changing the roles of whole departments in an institution. Often, a department whose activities are critical to profitability is precisely the department where management chooses to invest computer resources. Successful automation improves and integrates work processes and generates new management information that can ultimately cause the department to lose power it originally had. In the airline industry, for example, sophisticated computer systems for reservations and aircraft scheduling redistributed responsibilities and weakened the power held by reservations and scheduling departments.

In general, new information systems increase the power of high-level management by reducing ambiguity of performance, pinpointing responsibility, and providing analytical insight. Consequently, because top management has access to more data, the relative power of preparers of information at middle levels of management is weakened, since they are less able to unduly manipulate information for their own advantage.

This increased executive power often intensifies when, after implementing new information systems to provide new information, the executives of the institution rely on it for decisions of increasing impact—whether or not the system is equipped to adequately provide the necessary information. Once executives have come to depend on access to sophisticated information, they press for increasingly complex systems that, whether successes or failures, accelerate the need for even more investment in information systems.

Although computers may help institutions to change, the same computers, once installed, inherently inhibit change. They become cemented into the work processes of the institution and, like bricks and mortar, can't easily be dislodged. This problem will become more serious as computers, which were formerly located in one place, are used by growing numbers of departments and employees and are spread throughout the institution. Although this dilemma has no simple solution, top management can minimize the risk of debilitating error by selecting modern systems, controlling their evolution, and ensuring that competent, experienced information systems management is in place.

Information Technology: Challenge and Opportunity

Sound management techniques are the key to the successful use of information technology. Any institution seeking to implement comprehensive information systems faces a vast array of possibilities in choosing management methods and in managing a daily barrage of technological decisions. The CIO's crucial role is to manage and plan, to define problems and opportunities, and to set priorities for attention. Top management must be solidly and skillfully in control of an asset as important as information technology. In the past, institutions could choose to avoid use of complex computer technology, and their occasional use did not put the survival of the institution at risk. But, those experiences do not prepare us for the new era of business survival dependent on computer technology, just as the skills required for driving in small-town streets, where speed is curtailed and accidents are limited, do not prepare us for driving on the freeways of a large city, where unprepared for the competition and speed of other traffic, we could easily become a fatality.

Today, with fewer management levels and direct access to greater amounts of increasingly accurate information, executives are able to manage more effectively. Instead of scrutinizing and screening conflicting information, executives now may spend their time using the information to manage the institution. This leaner and more direct organizational structure, along with easy access to accurate information, provides new opportunities for productive management discussions of performance and results, and consequently improves the productivity and quality of the work of the institution.

Notes

1. W. R. Synnott and W. H. Gruber, *Information Resource Management* (New York: John Wiley and Sons, 1981), pp. 48–49, 66, 82–87.
2. P. Federico, *Management Information Systems and Organizational Behavior* (New York: Praeger Publishers, 1985), pp. 87–91.
3. B. F. Minard, "Growth and Change Through Information Management," *Hospital & Health Services Administration* 32, no. 3 (August 1987): 307–18.
4. Ibid.
5. P. Ein-Dor and E. Segev, *A Paradigm for Management Information Systems* (New York: Praeger Publishers, 1981), pp. 131–45.
6. Ibid.
7. Minard, "Growth and Change."
8. Ein-Dor and Segev, *A Paradigm.*
9. Synnott and Gruber, *Information Resource Management,* pp. 66–68, 325–29.
10. Federico, *Management Information Systems,* pp. 105–7.
11. Ein-Dor and Segev, *A Paradigm.*
12. B. F. Minard, "The Leadership Commodity," *CIO* (June 1988): 12–14.
13. F. W. McFarlan and J. L. McKenney, *Corporate Information Systems Management: The Issues Facing Senior Executives* (Homewood, IL: Richard D. Irwin, Inc., 1983), pp. 53–57.
14. Ibid., pp. 49–66.
15. Ein-Dor and Segev, *A Paradigm,* pp. 64–67.
16. Ibid., pp. 75–76.
17. Ibid., p. 142.
18. Ibid., p. 100.
19. B. F. Minard, "Modern Principles Improve Information Systems," *Healthcare Financial Management* (June 1988): 140–44.
20. Ein-Dor and Segev, *A Paradigm,* pp. 81–84.
21. Ibid., p. 50.
22. Ibid., pp. 64–67.

23. Ibid., pp. 94.

24. Minard, "The Leadership Commodity."

25. B. F. Minard, "Managing the Hospital's Portfolio of Information Systems," *Healthcare Strategic Management* 5, no. 1 (1987): 16–22.

26. Ibid.

27. Ibid.

28. C. Dunbar, "It's Not Me, It's We," *Computers in Healthcare* (Spring 1989): 17–20.

29. G. J. Mann, "Managers, Groups, and People: Some Considerations in Information System Change," *Health Care Management Review* 13, no. 4 (1988): 43–48.

30. Minard, "Growth and Change."

31. C. J. Austin, *Information Systems for Health Services Administration*, 3rd edition (Ann Arbor, MI: Health Administration Press, 1988), pp. 131–32.

32. F. J. Turisco and A. P. McMackin, "Leahy Clinic: Implementing an Order Entry and Result Reporting System for Cardiac Testing Using PCS/ADS," *Computers in Healthcare* (April 1989): 27, 30–32, 34.

33. J. G. Anderson et al., "Physician Use of HIS Impacts Quality of Care," *U.S. Healthcare* 6, no. 10 (October 1989): 41–42, 46.

34. D. H. McConnell and M. A. Brenner, "HIS: The Clinician's Role," *Computers in Healthcare* (June 1989): 20–22, 24.

35. D. J. Mishelevich et al., "Implementation of the IBM Health Care Support Patient Care System," in *Information Systems for Patient Care*, ed. B. I. Blum (New York: Springer-Verlag, 1984), pp. 62–82.

36. G. Kolenaty, "Hospital Information Systems Planning," in *Information Systems for Patient Care*, ed. B. I. Blum (New York: Springer-Verlag, 1984), p. 150.

37. L. W. DiGiulio and T. K. Zinn, "Actualizing System Benefits—Part III," *Computers in Healthcare* (July 1988): 26–28.

38. M. Malvey, *Simple Systems, Complex Environments* (Beverly Hills: Sage Publications, 1981), p. 51.

39. Ibid., pp. 13–14.

40. Ibid., p. 36.

41. A. G. Watlington, "Realizing System Benefits: Meeting the Implementation Challenges," *Computers in Healthcare* (May 1989): 28–29, 31–33.

42. A. G. Watlington, "Benefits Realization at Mercy Memorial Results in a Changed Organizational Culture," *Computers in Healthcare* (August 1989): 26–29, 32.

43. N. M. Lorenzi and E. B. Marks, "University of Cincinnati Medical Center: Integrating Information," *Bulletin of the Medical Library Association* 76, no. 3 (July 1988): 231–36.

44. Malvey, *Simple Systems,* p. 34.

45. J. G. Anderson et al., "Why Doctors Don't Use Computers: Some Empirical Findings," in *Use and Impact of Computers in Clinical Medicine*, ed. J. G. Anderson and S. J. Jay (New York: Springer-Verlag, 1987), p. 103.

46. Malvey, *Simple Systems,* pp. 156, 158, 174.

47. McFarlan and McKenney, *Corporate Information Systems Management*, pp. 17–18, 71.
48. M. Lundeberg et al., *Information Systems Development: A Systematic Approach* (Englewood Cliffs, NJ: Prentice-Hall, 1981), pp. 304–23.
49. Federico, *Management Information Systems*, pp. 87–91.
50. Ibid.
51. Minard, "Growth and Change."
52. Federico, *Management Information Systems*, pp. 100–103.

4

TECHNOLOGY: TELECOMMUNICATIONS, NETWORKING, AND INTERCONNECTED COMPUTERS

Telecommunications, networking, and interconnected computer systems, which currently represent the leading edge of information technology, hold the promise of improved efficiency and productivity through the sharing of work and data. Because these technologies provide the capability to use and share information in new ways both within the institution and outside the institution with individuals and other institutions, they offer great potential to health care institutions. They offer new ways to communicate and deliver clinical information, encourage the development of new work relationships, and can allow humans to team up to collect and use data to improve work flow in their institutions. Consequently, these technologies can provide a valuable competitive edge to health care institutions that use them to full advantage.

Reasons for Using Advanced Networks in Health Care

As more and more patient data are computerized and available to be retrieved from computer data bases, clinicians will press health care institutions for telecommunications and networking advancements that will allow them easy access to this data for support of their patient care activities. For example, Bryan Memorial Hospital in Lincoln, Nebraska, reports that their advanced telecommunications systems allow physicians to interconnect from their homes to the hospital information systems (HIS), gaining access to patient data and improving patient care.[1]

Advanced networking will allow orders, test results, and charge transactions to flow from the point at which the data are recorded to the ultimate destination without delay—and without moving through piles of paperwork from office to office and desk to desk—resulting in more accurate and timely patient charges, and fewer lost charges.[2] The advanced capabilities will allow innovation and redefinition of the logistics of the flow of data, eliminating many of the steps, and some of the complexity, imbedded in current systems for charge processing.[3]

Network interconnections can be established with relative ease among personal computer users for informal and infrequent sharing of data, such as files, and equipment, such as printers. At this fairly simple networking level, technology is available for transmitting messages and other information among users for work sharing and increased productivity. Interconnections can also be provided to exchange large blocks or entire files of data regularly and routinely. For example, patient charges may be passed from one computer to another on a daily schedule. In addition, unscheduled exchanges of data files for ad hoc processing can also be made, such as periodic downloading of HIS order entry work load statistics from the HIS to a personal computer in the physical medicine department for analysis using spreadsheet software.

At a more comprehensive level, network interconnections can be established to provide an integrated network of computer units specifically designed to facilitate employees' collective participation in departmental work. Such technology might be used in a radiology department to manage the tracking of films, to process orders, and to transcribe dictation into reports. At this networking level, computer units or terminals on the network can, in addition, gain immediate access to a minicomputer or mainframe computer to exchange patient data. Of course, this more sophisticated and integrated form of networking involves more complex technology. The necessity to protect data integrity during such data exchanges requires rigid logic that imposes a serial sequencing among potential simultaneous users of a specific data item, such as the data record of a patient's test result.

An even more complex capability automatically triggers a computer to send certain data to another computer. When a patient is admitted, for example, registration data are passed to all other computers requiring that data. The complexity of this process stems from each participating computer's need first to track any computer unable to receive data when originally sent and then to provide automated mechanisms that pass the data on when that computer rejoins the network.

Finally, the most sophisticated networking capability involves true cooperative, or more recently called, client/server processing. Here some processing takes place on one computer, the client; other requests are passed on to another computer, the server, for processing, with results returned to the client unit. Ironically, this capability is extremely complex precisely because it makes processing appear simple to the user. Within the information technology industry, terms like *seamless* and *transparent* indicate that the user at a workstation neither knows nor needs to know whether the computer's work is being performed by the desktop computer unit or by one of several interconnected computers.

Ultimately, high-speed, high-capacity computer networks will allow the transmission of computerized diagnostic images, such as those used in radiology or cardiology. These images, currently stored as physical images on radiology films, will be digitized and stored in computer files, and then immediately and simultaneously be available over networks whenever and wherever they are needed.

From Simple Interconnections to Computer Communities

In the mid-1970s, commercial interest in tightly interconnected computers emerged, survived for several years, and then expired. This capability was termed *distributed computing* initially, and more recently renamed *cooperative computing*. Proponents espoused the ability of data communications and networking technology to provide methods for interconnecting computer hardware, but they did not, however, adequately predict the difficulty of producing software and management methods to accomplish that feat. Furthermore, vendors and users alike failed to anticipate the formidable challenge of designing applications software that would function successfully in such a complex environment.

Networks have been used incidentally in the past in health care institutions to interconnect computers; today, however, the networks are as important a resource as the computers. Previously, only the most simple interconnections among computers were implemented. For example, large computers, usually called *mainframes*, were interconnected with one or several smaller minicomputers to exchange data about patient identification, patient location, and other important details. More recently, however, the proliferation of increasingly powerful desktop personal computers (PCs) has created a new challenge: how to make more effective use of PCs by interconnecting them with larger computers and with each other for cooperative computing, computers tightly coupled to share processing. This new wrinkle raises fresh technological issues about sharing information throughout an institution. It also adds yet another dimension to the already difficult challenge of managing a hospital's valuable information systems and data bases.

Initially, traditional methods of interconnecting computers required that large computers drive smaller computers. This called for the use of *emulation software* in the smaller computers so that the larger computer could be fooled into believing it was communicating with one of its family of terminals. In this master-slave relationship, no complex logic and, therefore, no useful sharing of work could be invoked in the data exchanges between the two components.

New methods for these types of interconnections have evolved over the past few years, and a sophisticated new peer-to-peer communication method has emerged: APPC (Advanced Program-to-Program Communication),[4] sometimes referred to by its abbreviated technical label, LU6.2. This new communications method allows computers, both large and small, to operate cooperatively as peers, allowing any one of several to tap one of the others on the shoulder, request data or cooperative processing, respond to a request, and automatically transfer its results. This type of interconnection will be quite valuable in consolidating the usefulness of several computers and bringing data from any of several computers to the workstation of a clinical professional.

Other new methods of communication have also emerged for the more complex interconnections among a group, or network, of computers in a local area, such as within a building or in adjacent buildings. Several alternatives provide for intercommunications within these local area networks (LANs). In one method, each computer in the network is allotted a brief time slice in which it and only it can tap another on the shoulder to conduct work. This method is similar to a child's game in which a token is passed around, and the holder of the token has a special privilege while it's in his or her possession. This method of gaining access to other computer units on the network is called the *token-passing media access method;* the network's electronics simulate the token possession and token-passing logic necessary to impose this turn-taking in the network.[5]

Another media access method uses logic very similar to the typical operation of CB radios that were popular a few years ago. In this method, a computer that needs to communicate with another simply broadcasts its communication on the network and then waits for a reply. If immediate interference from a simultaneous competing broadcaster is detected, termed a *collision* in this protocol, it simply broadcasts again, much like someone sending a message on a CB radio. This media access method, used in the family of

Ethernet networks, is called CSMA/CD (Carrier Sense Multiple Access with Collision Detection).

While there are many other media access methods and technical considerations, such as network topologies and transmission methods, the point here is to dramatize extremes and alternatives. At one extreme is a precise method of taking turns, designed to achieve a directed interconnection while attempting to optimize the network's capacity by providing a clear indication to the sending unit that the intended recipient did or did not receive the communication. At the other extreme is a trial-and-error method, subject to frequent resending of messages and using both network capacity and work of the interconnected computer units for detecting collisions and resending. Both these methods are widely used, and both are featured in products offered by many major vendors. Some vendors market products using both methods or variations of each.

Basic Concepts and Terminology

Just as information systems executives are learning to be comfortable in the language of the health care business, so should health care executives develop a working knowledge of the terminology of information technology. It is not necessary for health care executives to understand the electronics or computer languages involved, but a firm grasp of major issues will enable them to participate in planning decisions involving those issues.

Because technology has undergone great evolutionary upheaval within a short period, the emerging terminology of data communications and networking is so complex and ambiguous that even professionals in the field are only marginally able to communicate among themselves. The phraseology used to describe a myriad of technical alternatives includes acronyms and technical terminology that change daily. As a further impediment, jargon is sometimes used to conceal and disguise pertinent detail, often making the fine points so difficult to understand that listeners are discouraged from probing relevant issues. In short, the same newly emerging words are frequently used both by speakers who wish to express precise ideas and by speakers who intend to remain vague.

One of the earliest networking methods available uses telephone technology. Designed for voice traffic, telephone technology transforms the sounds of a person's voice into electronic analog signals that are then sent over thin copper wires (twisted-pair cabling or wiring). In this type of transmission, electronic signals are created (a process called *modulation*) with an amplitude proportional to the sounds and pitches of the person's voice, sent over the wires, and then transformed back into voice sounds and pitches at the receiving end.

When voice telephone transmission methods are used for data transmission, an additional level of transformation is required. The data are transformed first into sound signals, then transmitted over the phone lines just as voice traffic is transmitted. Then, at the other end, the sound signals must be transformed back into data.

Some local telephone companies are now installing modern equipment designed especially for data communication. This equipment relies directly on digital communication, using the computerized form of data as combinations of zeros and ones. In a computer, each data item, whether it is a numeric character, alphabetic character, or special symbol (for example, $, %, *), is first transformed into a unique combination of the numerals zero and one. Digital data communication, therefore, does not require the extra steps of transforming the zeros and ones first to sounds and then to analog signals; information is transmitted and received in its original digital form.

In fact, data communication and voice telephone communication technologies are gradually merging. Voice telephone communication, coming full cycle, is beginning to depend on digital communication methods: voice signals are converted to a stream of zeros and ones representing sounds and pitches.

It is this new digital communication technology that makes possible the cabling and transmission technology known as *fiber optics*. Instead of using copper wires for transmission, fiber optics technology uses fine strands of fiberglass through which light can travel. The resulting fiber optic cabling is much smaller and takes up less physical space than copper wires. Light is the medium for transmitting signals, and the presence or absence of light represents zeros and ones. This technology, essentially flashing a light on and off very rapidly, allows greater transmission accuracy and speed.

In addition to twisted-pair copper wire and fiber optics transmission media, the other major medium for data transmission is coaxial cable. This technology employs a signal similar to a cable TV signal and, like cable TV, can be implemented to transmit several simultaneous channels of signals, called a *broadband transmission*. When just a single channel is transmitted, it is called a *baseband transmission*.[6]

The transformation of numeric and alphabetic characters into codes composed of unique combinations of zeros and ones requires the existence of industry standards that all computer technology vendors accept. For example, the code for the letter *A* in one computer must be accepted as an *A* in another computer to which the code may be sent. Standards and conventions must also exist for special codes that are sent among computers for the purpose of starting and ending messages. Just as people may greet each other with a conventional "hello" before beginning a conversation, so must computers have such a convention. It is this variety of special codes and conventions that makes telecommunications technology so complex.

The earliest digital communication method, between computers and what were essentially teletype terminals, was *asynchronous* (not synchronized). In this method, a computer started transmitting without any knowledge of the teletype machine's readiness at the other end to receive a message. The teletype machine then transformed the combinations of zeros and ones into letters and numbers and printed them on paper.

Computers relying on the early, asynchronous transmission method had several disadvantages. They were incapable of allowing the receiving unit to request a retransmission necessitated by interference on those early telephone connections, which were much less reliable than they are today. To surmount these problems, a new, *synchronous* method was devised. It allowed a two-way synchronized exchange between sender and receiver, beginning with acknowledgments of readiness and receipt, and evolving over several years to incorporate more sophisticated error detection logic by which the receiving unit could sense possible errors and perform thorough checking on data it received.

Soon the complex combinations of hardware and software, together with the development of sophisticated synchronous data communication controls, required that new standards be established. In response to this need, IBM developed a new set of standards called Systems Network Architecture (SNA). This synchronous protocol included not only a new set of special codes, but also a hierarchy of seven data communications layers in which these codes would be used.[7]

In the lowest and most basic layer, a connection is established from hardware to hardware, and certain codes are exchanged between two hardware units to get them synchronized and ready to communicate. Once they are ready, the next layer, a software layer, then sends its code, like a "hello," and invokes a similar layer of software at the other end to respond with a greeting in return, signaling its readiness. At a higher layer, a more specialized software function might then send a code followed by a real message, such as a patient's name, from one computer to another. A similar layer of software on the other end must know what to do with that data. The APPC software described earlier is one example of software functioning at this higher layer. It has messages and codes recognizable by similar software at both ends of the transmission.[8]

Systems Network Architecture is fundamentally embedded in the software products of IBM, of vendors that use IBM products, and of vendors that have designed their products for compatibility with IBM products. With the growth and extension of this architecture, telecommunications technology has merged with computer technology.

More recently, the growth of networks and the emergence of other vendors' power to challenge IBM's influence on information technology standards and architecture have led to development of new architectures. One such architecture is the proposed Open Systems Interconnection (OSI) model, which, like SNA, has seven layers; however, it differs slightly in several of its layers, principally those involving networking.[9]

In either architecture, the processing of intermediate software layers governs the passing of data among networked computers. For example, the software at intermediate layers handles functions such as determining which network unit has the token, addressing the token to some other unit in the network, processing the acknowledgment, and essentially putting messages into electronic envelopes to send them to another unit. (No real token exists, of course; this concept simply describes the logic used to share a network.)

While it is at the top layers of software architecture that health care vendors' products provide the capability to perform hospital functions, such as registering a patient, it is at the lowest layers of the architecture that basic electrical operations take place. For these basic operations to succeed, the hardware and electronics at one end must be compatible with those at the other end. Referring back to the earlier example of analog and digital transmission over telephone lines, if an analog unit sends the signal, an analog unit must also receive it for any transmission to take place at that level and, therefore, at any higher level. Accordingly, if the sending unit is digital, the receiving unit must also be digital.

An additional characteristic of transmission in local area networks is topology, of which there are three basic types. In one topology, a *ring,* the networked computer units are connected in a closed ring. Alternatively, in a *star* topology, the units are connected to each other through one single unit at the center. The third type of topology, a *bus,* uses a simple linear link among the units, with no need for either a central unit or a closed loop.[10]

Each single local area network has a unique topology (for example, ring), transmission media (for example, twisted pair), signalling method (for example, baseband), and access protocol (for example, token passing). However, not all computer equipment is compatible with all combinations of topology, media, signalling, and access protocol.

In many cases, two networks using the same access protocols can be interconnected using a unit called a *bridge;* two networks using dissimilar access protocols can possibly be interconnected using a unit called a *router,* a combination of bridge and router (called a *brouter*), or a *gateway*. Unfortunately, not all dissimilar networks can be interconnected effectively.

These formidable stumbling blocks of incompatibility and complexity of interconnection have limited extensive use of networks. Incompatibilities exist not only in equipment, but also throughout intermediate software layers. For example, the highest layer of software for patient registration performs its telecommunications work through the six lower layers at both ends of the transmission. If a synchronous transmission is sent, that message cannot be received by an asynchronous terminal or by any other hardware or software product that does not have the proper intermediate layers. One great limitation of standard software is that most vendors' products, written at this highest layer, have not yet been enhanced to take advantage of the intermediate layers that provide networking protocols for links to computer units in networks.

The threat of obsolescence is another serious barrier to extensive use of local area networks. Rapidly changing products and a volatile computer technology market increase risks that an institution could select a hardware and software combination that will not endure in the market.

The proliferation of personal computer workstations is creating potential for new and enhanced applications, but at the same time it is also contributing to early product obsolescence. It has generated a growing market for new products, great change in those products, and consequently high risk and difficulty in making decisions in this dynamic environment. As a further consequence, installed products quickly are becoming obsolete.

These powerful forces are beginning to invade the previously more stable world of mainframe computers, minicomputers, and office automation. Local area networks are being developed to interconnect personal computer workstations not only with each other, for example, but also with the minicomputers and mainframe computers throughout an institution and outside its boundaries. These same forces are also accelerating the merging of office automation technology with computer technology. Such forces, plus myriad other powerful influences, threaten chances of success in selecting and managing telecommunications, local area networks, and cooperative computing strategies.

Available Products and Services

Computer, communications, and office equipment markets are slowly merging into one massive, consolidated market. Vendors are blending their products and services to maintain or develop strong market positions; in addition to simply offering their own products to many segments of the market, they are forming marketing partnerships, remarketing agreements, and other strategic alliances with other, sometimes competing, vendors. The resulting market spans an ever-widening range of products. It includes traditional mainframe and minicomputer hardware and storage devices, large printers and other equipment typically used in an institution's main computer center, and the systems software that enables this equipment to function. It also includes standard terminals, both video terminals and printers; connection devices such as modems; and data communications hardware and software that enable powerful computer equipment to connect with units outside the computer center. At the same time, a steady stream of new products, both hardware and software, is being introduced to interconnect these large computers to local area networks.

Many vendors now active in this market provide software designed for the health care industry. Some market hardware products as well as health care software that operates on their hardware. Software vendors usually provide software for a specific manufacturer's product. A software vendor might additionally be a remarketer (sometimes called a VAR, for *value added remarketer*) of the hardware vendor's equipment. Conversely, a major hardware vendor might market another vendor's software. In this case, the software product is sometimes renamed, even though it is the same product independently offered by another vendor. Similar combinations occur when software vendors obtain the rights to rename and integrate another software vendor's product into their own product line.

One segment of the overall market focuses on computerized telephone systems, called *public branch exchanges* (PBX) or *telecommunications switches*. These systems offer comprehensive new options to the telephone user, such as sophisticated conferencing alternatives, voice mail, and automated call-forwarding. They also offer possibilities for limited handling of data communications: connecting remote terminals or personal computers through the computerized telephone system to other computers could save the cost of routing other cabling to that location. Products and services in this market segment are provided by companies that were originally part of AT&T, as well as by several other specialized companies.

The particularly fast-growing market for personal computers and other desktop and small departmental computers is composed of several basic partitions. One family of computers, including IBM personal computers and compatibles, uses the DOS family of operating systems; other groups, which include Apple computers and computers that use the UNIX operating systems, do not. Memory capacity is another important characteristic differentiating personal computers. Older PCs based on the Intel 8088 chip, for example, are limited to a maximum memory of approximately 640,000 characters of memory; many newer PCs, however, have much larger memory capacities. Other variations in personal computers' internal speeds, disk storage capacities, and video screen capabilities also exist.

Another differentiation exists between computers that have the potential for processing multiple tasks (multitasking) and other, usually older, computers that cannot. The presence or absence of multitasking ability depends on the capability of the electronics circuitry (the chip) on which the computers are built. A computer built on an appropriate newer chip (such as the Intel 80286, 80386, or 80486) can potentially handle multiple tasks simultaneously if it also uses software with multitasking capability. These multitasking capabilities, which have been present in mainframe computers and minicomputers for many years, are now becoming available in small, desktop computers. Competing software products use the basic operating system families known as UNIX and OS/2, although there are variations of each.[11,12] These products are marketed by several vendors, and some vendors market both software families.

Word-processing software dominates the large and dynamic PC software market, with many vendors offering competing products. This market is especially volatile, however, because vendors continuously enter and leave the market. In addition, each vendor usually upgrades its products at least once a year. Consequently, customers should be wary of converting to a new word-processing product that magazine articles promote as the best; within a short time, similar existing products offered by competing vendors will likely be upgraded to include the same features.

Spreadsheet software for PCs is also very useful and popular, but only a few products have survived frequent market upheavals. This kind of software was originally conceived to do the work that an accountant does on a financial spreadsheet: arranging numbers in rows and columns, and adding across rows and down columns. But spreadsheet software is now being used to perform all sorts of office and departmental record keeping, such as keeping multicolumn lists and cross-referencing among columns of items, either numerically or alphabetically.

For office or departmental record keeping that cannot be accommodated using spreadsheet software, generalized data base software is now available for personal computers. However, only users who possess programming skills can take full advantage of this software's capabilities.

Software currently on the market allows personal computers to connect with other computers over telephone lines. Such software helps PCs emulate another piece of equipment in order to become compatible with software or hardware at the other end. This use of software for computer terminal emulation is one way to permit intercommunication among otherwise incompatible equipment, overcoming the problems discussed earlier in this chapter.

Another large market has recently developed for special equipment called *boards,* which were designed to allow personal computers to perform a range of functions, including emulation. A board contains electronic currentry that provides special enhancements. It is manufactured and marketed as a board intended for placement in a special slot inside the personal computer, and it is preprogrammed to work with the computer in which it is installed. Boards can provide a variety of special capabilities, such as extra computing power and additional internal computer memory.

One special-purpose board enables personal computers to operate on a local area network. Once the board is installed, the computer must also be equipped with software that can invoke the board's capabilities and, through it, gain access to other computers on the network.

A wide variety of products have been developed to perform networking and interconnection functions. *Protocol convertors* perform functions similar to the emulation capabilities already described, except that they function as intermediaries between otherwise incompatible products, translating from one protocol to another. Some vendors additionally provide networking equipment, such as amplifiers and routing equipment, and software that operates on this equipment to provide its capability.

The speed of telecommunications technology is increasing dramatically. In the early 1970s, the normal data transfer rate over a voice telephone line between a computer terminal and a computer was about 30 characters per second (a character is a number or letter, such as 0 or 1, A or B). Currently, similar data transfer achieves speeds of approximately 1,000 characters per second, 30 times faster, at equal or lesser cost than the earlier, slower rates. For a modest increase in cost, speeds of 2,000 characters per second can easily be accommodated; for a further cost increase, speeds of up to 6,000 characters per second can be reached over media available through telecommunications vendors such as the local telephone company.

Compared to telecommunications technology, networking technology is delivering even more dazzling speeds, up to approximately 400,000 characters per second. Although some of this capacity must be used for network management messages, the network's effective speed is still far more rapid than that of previous state-of-the-art telecommunications technology. Newer, slightly upgraded hardware and software technology will quadruple the 400,000 characters per second, and some research laboratories are beginning to reach speeds of six times that rate—or about 10 million characters per second. At these speeds, health care institutions may be able to transmit high-resolution diagnostic images over the network very quickly. As a result, networking of diagnostic images could soon become possible.

Personal computer workstations are becoming less costly and, at the same time, more capable. But the boards, other hardware, and interconnecting software are still costly and not yet as standardized as the basic hardware and software of PC workstations. Moreover, while local area networking media are improving and the speed of data transfer is increasing, software that makes comprehensive use of local area networking is not improving as quickly, and projects making use of this technology should be undertaken very cautiously, until it becomes more useful and reliable.

In addition to the great variety of products offered, the information technology market also includes a wide range of consultants to advise about hardware and software interconnections. Special consultants, sometimes called integrators, are available for assisting customers with intricate interconnections and integration of complex products provided by several vendors.

All vendors focus marketing strategies on their installed base of customers, the collection of current customers who are fairly well committed to use of that vendor's products. This installed base also includes customers of other vendors with which that vendor has marketing alliances. A vendor's marketing influence over its installed base preserves vendor products beyond their usefulness and usually ensures that a vendor's product remains differentiated from the rest of the market. This strategy prevents that vendor's products from blending well with other vendors' products and also prevents other vendors' products from blending with its products. This process sometimes keeps several product lines alive in the marketplace, even when one offers clearly superior technology. Once a customer is part of a vendor's installed base, shifting to other vendors' better products is extremely difficult and costly. Such a shift would require the customer to replace most hardware and software already installed and operating.

Vendors' tendencies to differentiate their products, preventing them from evolving toward other vendors' product lines, allows enterprising vendors to capitalize on unmet needs as an opportunity to establish a market niche. For example, a vendor may provide a slight variation of another vendor's product, a variation that customers can install as a substitute without great cost and difficulty. This substitute may provide the chance to blend with, and ultimately evolve to, a different technology. This approach is best exemplified by a personal computer manufactured to operate with both the DOS or UNIX operating systems. Such a PC lets customers continue to use current application systems based on DOS, but they can also easily evolve to new applications using the UNIX operating system.

The complex marketplace changes constantly as users and entrepreneurial investments create important new opportunities. For example, a new technological concept, such as an innovative new telecommunications method, may emerge and breed new vendor opportunities. One or more vendors may aggressively market new products incorporating the innovation. Users who believe that they have a need for the product become what the industry calls the "early movers." If the product is successful, it finds a niche in the market; other vendors then introduce similar products that are subtly enhanced. By the time a broad base of users understands the technology well enough to evaluate potential use and minor product differences, the market has shifted. Early products have become obsolete and are soon displaced by later products.

Analyzing Alternative Approaches and Selecting an Effective Strategy

The best place to begin the formidable task of selecting and planning networking technology is to consider the major technological, user, and management factors that affect selection, and to define objectives. Even though it may not be possible to achieve all objectives either immediately or with a single vendor product, objectives must be defined at the start of the process in order to choose the network technology that will best handle internal data communications traffic and, potentially, modest traffic volumes beyond the boundaries of the institution.

Factors that Affect Selection

Network selection activities are inherently complicated because they require at least some understanding of the complexities of past and present technologies.[13] And, unfortunately, the history of data communications is a litany of polarized strategies: at least two kinds of data encoding (cryptically labeled ASCII and EBCDIC), at least two types of sender-receiver synchronization (asynchronous and synchronous), and several generations of data transmission methodology. Additionally, the marketplace for data communications hardware and software is overflowing with marketing approaches that tend to complicate, rather than simplify, planning and selection processes.

The most important criterion in selecting technology usually is enough flexibility for future needs and requirements so that the technology will not become obsolete before the institution has realized a reasonable return on its investment of time and money. One workable approach involves planning for departmental local area networks that serve immediate and well-defined needs, such as the radiology department's needs, then later connecting these networks to a major corporate, or *backbone* network—a sort of universal data highway that links the smaller networks together. This strategy has the practical advantage of balancing long- and short-term objectives.[14] It satisfies immediate needs and gains immediate benefits, while at the same time creating a prototype to provide the institutional learning necessary for further planning. It is vital, however, to take particular care in selecting the departmental local area networks. Only those that are compatible with the technology planned for the corporate network will achieve future integration of functions and data. Vendors frequently attempt to convince departmental management that their products will magically interconnect and integrate with all future products. But many current local area network products do not interconnect well with all other products and, consequently, may be incapable of sharing in future corporate networks.

Ideally, the selected networking technology should be compatible with the collection of equipment, software, cabling, and procedures currently in use. It is also important that the technology, once installed, fit well with products, institutional requirements, and new information capabilities that the future will undoubtedly produce. In this era of rapidly changing networking technology, some possibility always exists that better, emerging products could eventually replace weak products currently installed. The best networking technology is compatible with the technological direction of these new products.

To prevent redundancy, software used as an integral part of the network should be compatible with other vendors' products. On the other hand, institutions should be cautious about planning to use vendors' software products that depend on integrated use of additional software from another vendor. Such a piecemeal combination sometimes creates unnecessary complexity and problems: the resulting marriage of products of two vendors may give inconsistent and unpredictable results, with neither vendor willing to assume responsibility for its successful use.

Flexibility for future use is crucial; therefore, choose technology that operates at the highest effective data speeds practical and that accommodates the higher speeds probable in the future. Such flexibility is important even though networking speeds may not be important for current networking use. If accounting professionals use a network for occasional access to shared data, for example, speed is not a critical factor in direct service to each user. However, if and when clinical users transfer large amounts of data, the speed of the network may be severely degraded, and other users' access may be limited.

The most desirable technology is planned so that units in the network operate as coprocessors or peers, not as masters and slaves. Furthermore, it is important that departmental computers be functionally part of the institutional network, unlike the stand-alone computers of the past era. In other words, departmental computers must not only technically connect, but also should participate in the controls and procedures that ensure necessary data integrity and the full advantages of integrated work. Such connections bring about the convergence of work processes that would otherwise be independent and possibly redundant. Failure to ensure the convergence of work processes can create added intellectual work in handling the problems of redundancy, ambiguity, or incompatibility.

Data security is a critical factor in all plans for providing broad data access or comprehensive data movement; network management therefore includes conventional access prevention and detection functions. Access controls can be planned and put in place to prevent unauthorized use of the network. Also, comprehensive controls over simultaneous access to files and records are sometimes necessary to control attempts at simultaneous data replacement in a single file by more than one computer. Data-tracking controls are additionally important, geared to provide reliable audit trails that can allow computerized reports showing who gained access to data and who updated stored data records.

Additionally, to ensure worker acceptance and workplace productivity, features available to the community of end users should not require knowledge of complex technical commands, but instead should be easy to use, preferably menu-driven.

Beyond Selection: Planning for the Network

A comprehensive networking plan specifies cabling and wiring that make use of wiring panels located in small, controlled utility rooms throughout the institution's buildings. Poorly managed cabling can be very expensive, not only because of material costs, but also because of expenses involved in hiring consulting architects, engineers, and electrical contractors to design conduits and cables that conform to fire and smoke control ordinances. Building-to-building and floor-to-floor wiring connections should be planned and precabled so that simple additions or changes can be made merely by plugging and unplugging wires in the wiring panels. Documenting wiring connections in a master reference guide, possibly in a computer system on a network, allows quick reference to those details as the network's operation is properly managed.

As the network evolves, the network plan can provide the potential for any terminal or personal computer to access any other computer in the network, under appropriate controls and using similar computer procedures and commands. For example, personal computers at nursing stations should be able to access both computers storing patient demographic data and computers storing clinical data, in addition to providing support of nursing unit record-keeping processes. Also, computers in physicians' offices, beyond the boundaries of the hospital, can be given similar access under appropriate data security controls.

Managing a Network

Comprehensive network management functions must be included and available so that performance measurement and rapid failure diagnosis are possible, including high-quality controls for preventing failure and for diagnosing, isolating, and recovering from network problems.

Administration

Good network administration and management methods ensure that the network is an institutional asset instead of an uneconomical and marginally useful liability. Toward this end, it is vital that the institution be able to solve network problems and define and implement network reconfigurations quickly and easily.

One important administrative responsibility is the careful documentation of the locations of networking equipment. Thorough documentation covers all the connected units and includes up-to-date specifications on cabling paths that link the equipment in networks, with cross-references designating which equipment is connected to each network. This documentation strategy reduces costs because equipment may be reconfigured without requiring vendors' expensive assistance.

Similar documentation of the versions of installed networking software is also basic to sound network management. It also may be wise to designate special naming conventions for files shared among network users so that similarly named files and misunderstandings about file names do not lead to confusion or even network failure. Special procedures for backup of network files can become an administrative issue unless this responsibility is delegated to specific network users. And no matter how simple the network is to use, training is always a necessary ongoing activity.

Diagnosis, Repair, and Recovery

Successful networking depends on good methods for diagnosing problems, detecting and isolating faults, repairing malfunctions, and recovering from failure—methods that ensure the network's reliability and efficiency. These methods could involve keeping emergency replacements for some critical equipment on hand. At the least, designated staff will need access to comprehensive diagnostic tools that they can use to locate network problems or sense degrading functions quickly. Such tools, however, cannot depend on the network's successful operation; otherwise, if part of the network is inoperable, the diagnostic tools could be useless.

Monitoring and Statistics

Monitoring procedures and tools provide effective means to gather valuable performance statistics on network operation. Maintaining statistics for such functions as traffic loading and timing delays at certain nodes on the network allows both measurement of performance and monitoring of traffic trends. Insight gained from such monitoring allows the network manager to plan reconfigurations that eliminate bottlenecks, fine-tuning the system and avoiding added costs of additional capacity. Monitoring can also detect unusual and unexpected traffic and, therefore, sense faulty software operation or users' incorrect practices. Careful analysis may additionally lead the network manager to define usage controls and limitations on some software in order to prevent future network traffic problems.

Diverse Network Uses

Integrated use of diverse hardware and software in a network results in a complex web of network traffic that requires careful management. Network traffic includes not only simple, short-duration traffic, such as frequent computerized patient test results sent from one computer to another, but also periodic transfers of large blocks of data from one user workstation to another. Some network software efficiently directs messages and data specifically to another unit on the network; other, less mature software may use the network less efficiently. Similarly, some users may be skillful enough to use the network competently; other users, who invoke software processes that send redundant data or otherwise use the network inefficiently, should be subject to network management controls.

Access security and data confidentiality also require careful management and control. The potential for integrated and simultaneous network use, with valuable corporate data moving through the network, makes data security issues a major concern for the network manager.

Another management concern involves imposing controls to prevent and detect invasions of software viruses—small programs typically embedded and hidden in other programs passing into or through a network. Software viruses are typically created as pranks by outsiders, but they could just as easily be conceived and inserted by disgruntled employees. Such a hidden program can be invoked when an unsuspecting user starts up a computer each day, unknowingly providing means for the unauthorized program to operate and allowing it to spread further or perform some unauthorized operation. As pranks, such programs usually produce some surprise (frequently a special message on the video screen), but they can also insidiously destroy or corrupt great amounts of valuable data.

One of the most challenging network management issues is the management and control of a growing investment in the network as an information technology asset. Technical complexity has escalated to the point where information technology problems that once were obvious management issues are increasingly abstract and ambiguous and, consequently, far more difficult to detect, manage, and control. In the past, for example, when an employee improperly used an important resource such as medical supplies, management processes detected the faulty practice, triggered corrective action, and controlled the potentially rising cost. In the abstract and complex world of modern information technology, however, nebulous and abstract resources, such as disk storage space or computer capacity, for example, may be routinely misused without detection because management's ability to pinpoint and correct the misuse is much more limited.

To counter these wasteful practices, the network manager can devise methods that make networking assets more subject to review, more controllable, and more manageable. Imposing a monthly capacity reporting system, for instance, would automatically create some restraints on haphazard use of these valuable resources.

Future Evolution and Trends

Compatibility: Health Industry Interconnection and Interfacing Standards

Many of the software and hardware products currently available are incompatible for interconnection and integration on networks; if they were more compatible, information technology would be less costly and more usable to the health care industry. Product prices are inflated because hardware and software must be redundantly tailored to interconnect and exchange data with other vendors' products. Likewise, incompatibility means that installation and implementation of vendor products require expensive additional effort, while system operation and maintenance are more difficult and costly because of awkwardness and poor interconnections among the products.

To eliminate this incompatibility in the future, health care information systems vendors must rethink their approaches to design and marketing. They must accept the fact that a single vendor cannot meet all the information technology needs of the health care industry—or even of a single health care institution—and they must work together to define industry standards. Simple standards, such as for the maximum number of characters to be reserved in the system for a patient's name, must be defined and consistently implemented in all vendors' products. Standards for passing data among computers also cry out for definition, so that various products from different vendors will fit together to meet health care industry needs at a lower cost. A special committee of the Institute of Electrical and Electronics Engineers (IEEE), the MEDIX (Medical Data Interchange) Committee, is currently working on standardization of medical data exchange among software and hardware products.[15] As a result of this and other efforts to promote and develop standards, more cost-effective information technology options eventually will become available.

Portability: Software that Operates Anywhere in the Network

Computer programs written for one family of computers usually do not operate on a computer from a different family of computers. This incompatibility stems not so much from hardware differences, but from operating system and other system software differences. Consequently, an institution that attempted to replace a computer with a more powerful model would, in many cases, find that currently functioning software would not operate, even with slight modifications, on the new computer. Likewise, software that is moved from one department to a department that uses a different computer probably will not operate on that computer.

Computer languages and system software tools must be transformed so that a computer program written for one computer can be moved to operate on another computer. Software programs must be partitionable, for example, so that some parts of the software can operate on computers other than the one from which a function may be invoked. Partitioned parts may even dynamically be allocated to operate on any one of several alternative computers, depending on which is available and suited to the task.

In answer to these needs, some major vendors are now undertaking comprehensive, multiyear efforts to establish a new, more flexible architecture. One of these new-generation architectures is called Systems Application Architecture (SAA).[16]

Simultaneous Use: Multiuser Personal Computer Software

The personal computer revolution initially promised great productivity by making computers available to health care personnel at their desks, allowing them to perform tasks better and faster than the tasks could be performed manually. To fulfill that promise, the industry initially delivered word processing and spreadsheet software. Now, networking hardware and software is allowing transition to a new era that will offer opportunities for several people to work together on one activity by using multiuser software through networks.

Multiuser software allows a single personal computer to work on several tasks concurrently, thereby serving several processes simultaneously. Emerging networking software is incorporating this concept to allow people at several computer units to work cooperatively, possibly directing results to each other or collecting data from each other. Additionally, any unit on the network can also invoke the processing of a distant computer that another unit is using at the same time. For example, powerful data base management software resident in one computer is able to grant access for input and retrieval of data from many other computers, even while the computer is in use. Multiuser software allows work to be better partitioned among people, letting professionals delegate and share their work with support staff.

Speed, Capacity, and Storage: Diagnostic Images

Much of health care's diagnostic information is stored in the form of images, such as those used in radiology and cardiology. Manual access to physical files of these images is labor-intensive and, as a result, subject to data loss and other potential problems that ultimately prevent quick access. Consequently, health care providers are often delayed and frustrated in their efforts to obtain and use this information when and where they need it to provide patient care.

If diagnostic images were computerized, they would be immediately and simultaneously available anywhere they were needed. However, if diagnostic images are to be computerized, they must first be transformed into ones and zeros representing the rows and columns of tiny dots that make up a single image, and there is some risk that the quality of transmitted images could be poorer than that of originals. Image quality depends on how many tiny dots are created from the original; to maintain quality, the number of dots should be as high as possible. On the other hand, this large quantity of dots represents an even larger quantity of ones and zeros that the computer must to store and transmit. As discussed earlier in this chapter, data transmission speeds and capacities will soon increase enough to handle these large volumes of data. But great volumes of data require costly disk storage devices to permit quick retrieval, and such storage would not be cost effective using the magnetic disk storage technology currently in use for on-line access. Emerging optical disk storage technology and other high-density storage devices, however, may provide new opportunities to store large volumes of data less expensively.

Continuity: Comprehensive Cooperative Computing Is Here to Stay

The cooperative computing concept first emerged in the mid-1970s, but the computer industry failed to deliver the capability necessary to transform the concept into reality. Since then, however, the advent of major enhancements in computer processing speed, data communications maturity, and networking capabilities have repositioned us for a new focus on this concept. We have also vastly improved our collective professional competence and management expertise. Even more importantly, health care's needs for enhanced information systems are driving us inescapably toward networking and cooperative computing. Spurred by the introduction of personal computers, employees and physicians are beginning to anticipate information availability that they would not even have imagined possible just a few years ago.

Networking and cooperative computing have arrived—and this time, they are here to stay. Computers can stay in touch: automatically exchanging critical patient data, consolidating them with other data, and formulating information that might not have existed otherwise. Networking will provide efficient, flexible, and manageable linkages that can be used to exploit opportunities for improving relationships and cooperation between clinicians performing related activities. Networking is no longer only a technological challenge for technologists. And management control of networking is not simply a convenient apron string for gaining conformance over computer users. It is an opportunity for an important strategic advantage. Health care institutions must grasp this critical opportunity by undertaking comprehensive technological planning for modern networks of interconnected computers and data integration. Because the technology is complex, it may require several years and phases to achieve significant progress.

Health care management stands at a critical crossroad, with a pressing need both for mature information technology and for leadership in providing that technology at a reasonable cost. Interconnections among information systems are critical to management; therefore, top management must control the planning for information technology throughout the health care institution. These information networks are the highways over which data pass from computer to computer, from video terminal to computer, and to and from the world outside the institution. They are as crucial to modern health care institutions of today as the railroads were to American industry in the past century.

Notes

1. L. Martin, "Anytime, Anywhere Healthcare," *Computers in Healthcare* (July 1989): 51–52.
2. W. P. Pierskalla and D. Woods, "Computers in Hospital Management and Improvements in Patient Care—New Trends in the United States," *Journal of Medical Systems* 12, no. 6 (1988): 426.
3. J. A. Wesley, "It Started with the Cow Path: Working Flatter, Not Faster," *Computers in Healthcare* (October 1989): 28–30.
4. IBM Corporation, *An Introduction to Advanced Program-to-Program Communication: APPC,* Document GG24-1584, 1987.
5. S. Tompkins, "Productivity Improvements for the Knowledge Worker: Personal Computers on Local Area Networks," presented at the ECHO (Electronic Computing Health Oriented) Fall Conference, 1987.
6. Ibid.
7. G. W. Goraline, *Computer Organization: Hardware/Software* (Englewood Cliffs, NJ: Prentice-Hall, 1986), pp. 596–97.
8. IBM Corporation, *An Introduction.*
9. R. A. Edmunds, *The Prentice-Hall Encyclopedia of Information Technology* (Englewood Cliffs, NJ: Prentice-Hall, 1987).
10. Tompkins, "Productivity Improvements."
11. Peter Birns et al., *UNIX for People* (Englewood Cliffs, NJ: Prentice-Hall, 1985).
12. M. S. Kogan and F. L. Rawson, III, "The Design of Operating System/2," *IBM Systems Journal* 27, no. 2 (1988): 90–104.
13. B. F. Minard, "The Rebirth of Distributed Computing in a Hospital Setting," *Healthcare Computing and Communications* (February 1987): 54–58.
14. F. W. McFarlan and J. L. McKenney, *Corporate Information Systems Management: The Issues Facing Senior Executives* (Homewood, IL: Richard D. Irwin, Inc., 1983), p. 48.

15. Institute of Electrical and Electronics Engineers, Medical Data Interchange Committee, IEEE Standards Project #1157, MEDIX, minutes of September 6, 1988, meeting.
16. E. F. Wheeler and A. G. Ganek, "SAA: Introduction to Systems Applications Architecture," *IBM Systems Journal* 27, no. 3 (1988): 250–63.

5

TECHNOLOGY: PERSONAL COMPUTERS AND END-USER COMPUTING

Giving Users Direct Access to Information Technology

The technologies covered in this chapter are important not so much because they are new and on the leading edge of information technology, but because they provide the means by which health care end users, the ultimate users of the information acquired through information technology, can gain direct access to computers and their data. End-user computing, together with the advances in networking technology discussed in Chapter 4, will allow physicians and nurses to use information technology closer to where patient care is provided.

End-user tools available on large computers take the form of user languages for retrieving information, performing analyses, and producing reports. Driven by consumer demand and vendor competition, the capabilities of these tools are advancing rapidly.

More recently, personal computers have become a major force in advancing and shaping end-user computing. Equipped with menu-driven software, they offer powerful, user-oriented capability directly to users. Easy-to-use personal computer software packages for word processing and spreadsheets, along with easy-to-use programming packages such as the dBASE product line, provide valuable capabilities that large mainframe computers have not been able to match.

End-User Computing on Large Computers

Computer technology was first used in health care to perform clerical and accounting functions. Computers next found favor as a way to automate an enterprise's operational transactions. These early computers required accounting and business office users to transcribe data onto forms and then send batches of these forms to the data entry department, where the data were entered onto punched cards (or, later, tape or disk media). Meanwhile, users awaited the scheduled processing of the information and subsequent computer-printed reports of results. Advancing technology eventually offered on-line access: video terminals that provide direct computer access to people, such as accountants, in the working environment.[1] Ultimately, much of the data entry and some information inquiry activity were converted to make use of on-line access by workers at the point of patient care or other point of work in departments throughout the hospital.

At the same time, as more and more operational transactions of the hospital were becoming automated, more and more data were being printed in reports. Content and format of these computerized reports were defined by middle-level managers and supervisors, and each report usually contained information required by a single department, such as the payroll department. Copies of those reports were typically passed up through the management ranks. Because each department has a vested interest in feeding certain information upward through the management hierarchy, high-level managers were inundated with reports—and they were forced to wade through an avalanche of data for the information they sought. As a result, managers became interested in extending on-line data inquiry capability to provide information retrieval of selected summary data and to perform some data analysis. This interest gave birth to a range of products, including *user report writers*, that allowed users at their terminals to produce reports fairly quickly and without complex programming. Additionally, data base products such as data dictionaries were developed and improved for quick and easy use with end-user on-line products.

User report writer technology was eventually extended to include generalized *user inquiry languages*. These languages allow the direct presentation of analytical and summary data on the video terminal, as opposed to presenting the data in paper reports that are printed elsewhere. Gradually, new and more advanced user inquiry languages were developed, through which users could obtain more data at their terminals. A new term, *decision support systems*, was coined to describe these tools, which support management by enabling them to access and analyze data for solving unstructured problems—problems for which no reports or data analyses patterns had previously existed.[2] Decision support system capabilities became useful in management analyses, financial analyses, marketing analyses, productivity analyses, case-mix analysis, retrieval of clinical data for use in patient care, and in data retrieval for medical research.[3]

Despite great effort and investment, however, acceptable capability simply did not materialize. Products were continuously unable to satisfy the pressing need for easy user access to the data. Eventually, user inquiry languages were improved to include English-language phrases. Some, dubbed *executive support systems,* used words such as *find, select,* and *calculate,* together with data dictionaries that included words like *patient, physician, department,* and *revenue.* Even these languages, though, did not meet the ultimate test: they were not easy enough to use to gain hands-on acceptance from such targeted end-user decision makers as managers, executives, nurses, physicians, and medical technicians. Assistance from staff analysts, skilled in the use of these languages, was almost always necessary, thus limiting the usefulness of the system capabilities.

Other major problems hindered early efforts to provide comprehensive end-user computing capabilities. One stumbling block was the computer software industry's inability to define and develop the software products needed for this market. In fact, creating such software products would have been nearly impossible during the technology's infancy. Users' growing computer literacy and changing expectations created a constantly changing market, changing technology and experts' changing theories continuously shifted the technological approach, and project management difficulties and budget overruns limited the ability to provide the end-user products desired.

In addition, end-user computing required enormous processing capability of the computer. Extensive and costly computer power was necessary for such functions as interpreting and translating the English words of user languages (for example, SELECT ALL PATIENTS WITH DRG 108) into computer instructions, checking the user language's special grammatical rules, detecting errors and providing error messages, and—finally—executing the instructions. All told, billions of computer instructions must be executed to translate the user language into the ones and zeros of computer instructions, and billions more are ultimately required to execute the instructions.

Changes Brought by Personal Computers

Early Word Processing

At the same time that end-user computing was developing on large computers, the personal computer emerged—literally out of the garages of early enthusiasts. These first personal computer units had very little internal memory, barely enough for the smallest programs to operate, and had very primitive system software. The early units had no disk or diskette drives. Instead, data and programs were loaded and stored using magnetic tape media equipment, very similar to that used in tape recorders and tape playing units.

During this period, the market for word-processing office equipment was also changing. Word-processing office equipment had been in use for several years, incorporating computer-like equipment the size of large office furniture and operated by centralized word-processing departments. These gave way to dramatically smaller desktop word-processing units that were electronically very much like the emerging personal computers.

A word-processing software package, WordStar, soon emerged for the personal computer, and this software became so popular that the market began comparing its capability favorably with that of the era's mature word processors. WordStar brought the similarity between word-processing equipment and personal computers into clearer focus.

Dramatic Technological Growth and the Emergence of New Vendors

The capability of personal computers grew rapidly and was eventually improved to provide data storage on diskettes, include greater amounts of memory, and use an operating system called CP/M (Control Program for Microcomputers). Other major hardware and software vendors soon entered the market. One of the largest, IBM, christened its personal computer the PC. Working together, IBM and Microsoft, a software vendor, created a new operating system, DOS (Disk Operating System).

Spreadsheet Software

Finally, spreadsheet software emerged as the first powerful analytical product for end-user computing on personal computers. An early product, Visi-Calc, stimulated growth in the personal computer market. Accounting departments of health care institutions quickly made use of spreadsheet software; to prepare financial reports, accountants could now enter rows and columns of accounting numbers into files while the totals were automatically calculated. Spreadsheet software was especially useful in analyses of proposed increases in charges for services because it could quickly calculate and present the expected results of the price changes. The great value of spreadsheet software is that it provides the capability to perform block functions, such as moving entire rows and columns, or to perform arithmetic computation on all data items in a block, such as increasing all values in a column by a given percentage.

Spreadsheet applications grew beyond accounting and soon were used to perform similar data presentation and analysis functions on other types of lists in accounting departments, as well as in other departments such as the medical records department and nursing departments. Other spreadsheet software products, such as Lotus 1-2-3, followed, offering greater capability. At the same time, new data base products emerged, such as those from dBASE, which provided better functions for analyzing data, especially large data bases of clinical data (for example, analysis of charges for all renal cases of a given month).

Stimulated Use of PCs by Innovative Support Departments

Meanwhile, information services departments in some hospitals devised an innovative method of providing support for end-user computing. They created the *information center,* where one or more employees fluent in end-user languages were specifically assigned to advise, guide, teach, and offer one-on-one assistance to employees of other hospital departments. Although originally created to support users of mainframe software, the information center concept eventually expanded to support personal computer users as well.[4]

Continuing the Frantic Evolutionary Pace

Personal computer technology "has become an integral part of—if not the major impetus behind—the phenomenon of end-user computing."[5] Personal computers provide raw computing capacity that is, in terms of how many instructions can be performed per second, much cheaper than that provided by large computers. This economy results principally because personal computers do not require the same complex internal electronics and software needed to handle a large computer's great variety of internal computer functions. And even if that processing capacity is used inefficiently by the end-user computing software, no simultaneous user is adversely affected because the personal computer is being used only by the user seated at the workstation.

In addition, software for personal computers is easier for vendors to develop, primarily because programs for personal computers are simpler to write than those for large computers. As a result, the range of software products being developed for personal computers is far wider than what might have been developed for large computers over a similar period of time with similar resources. Consequently, software for personal computers is usually far less costly than for large computers.

Meanwhile, the volatility and unpredictability of the end-user software industry continue to accelerate at an increasingly brisk pace. Today, the capabilities of end-user computing are evolving rapidly in the same trial-and-error fashion as did end-user computer products for larger computers. Products are continually being displaced by new models with new capabilities as a tremendous thrust for innovation is driven by users' requests and market competition. In the earliest days of overlapping waves of product changes and new products, corporate assets at risk were limited. Later-model personal computers, for example, could easily be justified to displace the few units purchased by the hospital a mere few months earlier, and the earlier units could be transferred to other users within the hospital. Similarly, with only a small number of personal computers installed, the investment in several copies of an early software package could be easily written off when a more capable package was available. But some hospitals now have installed hundreds of computers, and they have invested significant assets in purchasing and learning to use early software products.

Furthermore, the integration of many software products into complex interdependencies prohibits easy implementation of changes and further complicates the issue. More recently, the advent of networking has created an additional wave of interdependencies that further compound the problem. Obviously, we are at the end of an era of simple decisions and inexpensive options, and we are entering a time fraught with the danger that this new technology, if not properly planned and managed, could lead to costly chaos.

End-User Computing in Health Care

End-user computing can bring tremendous capability to clinical processes to reduce costs and improve quality. The technology of networking, plus new, more reliable methods for interconnection among computers for data integration, and new easier-to-use languages for retrieval and analysis, collectively make clinical productivity enhancements possible.

The technology will reduce waiting times for orders, test results, and other information. Since it will allow data entry and retrieval closer to the point of care, it will allow a reduction in data errors. And it will make the clinicians more productive, both because they have easier access to data and also because the analytical capabilities of end-user computing will complement their skills and knowledge. Clinicians will have, for example, access to data analysis software, graphical presentations, and ultimately, "expert systems" software that will compare data against norms, check interdependencies among drugs, and also check interdependencies between specific drugs and laboratory test results and patients' allergies and sensitivities.[6]

More and more physicians are becoming comfortable with end-user computing techniques, and many have reached high levels of proficiency; medical schools have courses on these topics, and many professional societies actively promote professional papers and symposium papers on these topics.[7]

Some clinicians believe that as end-user computing capabilities advance, physicians and nurses will become the primary users of information technology in health care, displacing the physician staff assistants, nursing secretaries, and other administrative people.[8] They believe that only when the caregivers can use the technology themselves will efficiency, productivity, and quality gains be realized and the computerized medical record be achieved, since only then will the data accuracy, consistency, and relevance be such that the resulting computerized medical record will be useful. Computerized nurse charting, for example, had been in place at LDS Hospital in Salt Lake City for two years when a study of physician acceptance found that "75% indicated that they considered the patient data to frequently or always be more accurate than the paper chart," and "66% believed that it frequently or always took them less time to locate data in the computer as compared to the paper chart."[9]

Tools for End-User Computing Today

End users currently have a variety of tools at their disposal. Usually, a desktop video display unit is connected to a computer that provides the capability to access data independently and perform functions needed to accomplish assigned work. The desktop unit typically contains, or is located near, a computer processor. The video unit, or monitor, usually has sharp graphics. The library of available software includes the capability to present high-quality graphics on the screen or on paper using a nearby graphics printer. The library of capabilities may be specialized, for example, to the needs of a particular department such as the cardiology department, or it may be sufficiently broad to include word processing, spreadsheet software, data base software, statistical analysis software, and computer programming languages. The desktop unit has extensive capability for accessing data bases and for storing data temporarily on disks—either in the local computer unit or in a more centralized disk storage facility. A user may share work and data with other users or may gain access to the data and functions of larger corporate computers.

The Marketplace for End-User Computing Tools

As mentioned in Chapter 4, the computing, telecommunications, and office automation markets are merging and consolidating; they are becoming broader and are growing in several directions. All three of these industry markets provide products that contribute to advancing end-user capabilities.

Many new products entering the market have achieved great success, such as Lotus 1-2-3. In fact, the potential payoff from investment in new products is so great that venture capitalists are actively seeking opportunities to participate in new ventures. This influx of venture capital and the resulting competition for market position are additional major forces accelerating the pace of innovation, change, and the emergence of new products. Growth is so rapid, in fact, that many products become obsolete shortly after they reach the market.

Essentially, two market segments support end-user computing. One segment provides products to support end-user computing that relies on the data bases and functions of large computers. The other segment provides products that support end-user computing on personal computers. Let's examine these two segments individually.

Products and services that operate on large computers

All end-user products provide some sort of easy-to-use language that professionals and managers can use while seated at a computer terminal. Users enter specific commands in the language to enter data into and retrieve data from data bases, perform some analysis on that data, and then present that information either directly on the screen, on a nearby printer and graphics device, or both. As users review the results of their work, they may reconsider and modify or extend their comments, and review the new results.

Some software products provide only the language, its special grammar rules, and its special utility functions, such as the capability to store a request and invoke it later to access other data—all without having to enter the specifics of the request again. In these software products, the user language works independently of the data base software, or even the specific computer hardware, operating behind the scenes. The language involved can be used with any of several data base structures. One such language is called structured Query Language (SQL), a universal language that is available with many vendors' data base products in the health care industry. A language possessing this characteristic usually becomes widely used in the industry, evolving and growing with use.

Other software products provide a powerful data base software package in addition to the user language. This type of combined software is usually more efficient in its use of computer resources, but it usually also has more limited capability. The life span of such a software product depends in large part on the vendor's continuing research, development, and marketing. For lack of this kind of continuous vendor support, many products have come and gone in this market segment.

Personal computer products and services

Computer processing units. Personal computer processing units are growing in capability and simultaneously becoming less costly. The cost decrease is driven by economies of scale (producing and marketing greater numbers of units) and by the competition resulting when the computer unit itself is subject to commodity pricing pressures. Furthermore, because the price of the computer unit is more visible than that of related products, vendors price it as low as possible, inducing prospective customers to buy, while banking on the greater profits they will derive from subsequent purchases of software and equipment. The costs of specialized boards and other supporting equipment, for example, remain fairly high, primarily because they are growing more complex.

The processing speeds of computer processing units, measured in MIPS (millions of instructions per second), now rival those achieved by mainframe computers of just a few years ago. Recently, a new type of computer technology called RISC (Reduced Instruction Set Computing), which is less expensive to manufacture, is beginning to bring about similar reductions in the cost of manufacturing personal computer workstations. At the same time, internal personal computer memory, which just a few years ago was measured in thousands of characters and limited to approximately 640,000 characters in personal computers using DOS, now is available in millions of characters—again rivaling what is available from mainframe computers. Moreover, disk drive capacity, measured in millions of characters and limited to five to ten million a few years ago, is now available in hundreds of millions of characters, and is also approaching the capacity available in mainframes.

Computer processing units are available from several manufacturers, such as Apple, Compaq, and IBM, in many models. One of the main differences in computer processing units offered by competing manufacturers is the internal method of moving data around inside the personal computer. Data are sent internally from place to place in a special internal pipeline, known as a *bus*. Different manufacturers use different bus technologies, and some even employ different bus technologies within their own different products. These differences in bus technologies are important because manufacturers of support equipment, such as those constructing boards, incur a greater expense in building a range of support components compatible with each of the different bus technologies, which in turn increases the price to the consumer.

Video display units. Cost reductions and improvements in the capabilities of video display units are being similarly accelerated by technological progress. Graphic presentation provides increasingly better video screen resolution and sharper images, and the technology for producing high-quality color images is advancing at a great pace. Some manufacturers, such as Apple, have gained substantial market position by leading the industry in advancing the usefulness of high-quality video graphics and images.

Printing technology. Printing has shifted from impact technology to many other forms, such as laser printing. These new methods offer a more letter-quality appearance, high-quality graphics integrated in documentation material, a variety of fonts and type sizes within a single document, reduced operating noise, and speedier printing. Because these newer technologies are less mechanical, they also are more trouble free than earlier methods. Here again, some manufacturers, such as Hewlett Packard, have gained considerable market share by leading the industry in laser printing.

Operating system software. Operating system software has evolved continuously. Early versions required the entry of coded commands to direct the system. A user who wanted to copy a file, for example, was required to enter the word COPY, followed by a very precise series of letters and symbols that designated disk drive units and abbreviated names of files, punctuated by commas, colons, slashes, and blank spaces. If the sequence or spacing of the letters and symbols was incorrect, the computer provided very little help diagnosing the error or instructing for correction. In newer versions, commands have been replaced by menus (lists of choices), or icons (pictures of choices) which users use to select among choices that specify the desired processing. Also, much better diagnoses and instructions are provided in response to errors. Later versions of operating system software offer networking capabilities, greater efficiency of internal work, faster access to data, and improved error detection.

Future development will provide even greater improvement in these functions. We can also expect to see better capabilities for using very large programs and data files, along with improved data presentation on the video screen. Future operating system software (OS/2 and newer versions of the

UNIX family of software) will also provide important extensions of the capability to simultaneously process more than one activity.

Application software. Software that provides specialized usage beyond that offered by system software is known as *application software* because of its application to the work of institutions. Application software capability has historically lagged behind that of hardware and operating system software.

Currently, however, growth in the application software field is taking three major directions. One avenue of growth continues the direction of the past: the search for new record keeping processes to be used on personal computers as they are used to automate more processes in hospitals. The health care industry, for example, is increasingly using bar code technology with personal computers to help record and control inventory and usage of materials and equipment throughout many departments. Bar code labels are being placed on supplies, medications, patient's identification bracelets, employee identification badges, clinical equipment, and furniture.

The second direction of growth is a continuing effort to upgrade existing application software in parallel with, and taking advantage of, the increased capabilities of hardware and operating system software. Word-processing, spreadsheet, and data base software packages, for instance, are being revised to take advantage of new capabilities for handling greater volumes of data or for accommodating new video screen capabilities.

The third area of application software growth is in ease of use. Graphics and other video techniques are greatly improved by the use of graphic user interfaces (GUIs) and *windows* on screens. Windows provide a means for partitioning the video display so that the background remains in place and a small window of information is superimposed on it. Graphic user interfaces provide improved screens and screen pointers to permit easier choice among processing options. For example, users may simply point at icons on the screen by touching the screen with a finger, light pen, or other pointing device, instead of selecting from a wordy menu.

Communications and networking. Communications and networking improvements are gradually providing work- and data-sharing capabilities that are being used, in turn, by application software to enable workers at different computers to manipulate data from the same data bases. Similar advancements also provide improved software for electronic mail—the communication of messages among users of a network. This enhanced software allows users to send electronic mail to electronic mail boxes and provides addressees automated options for retrieving, reading, forwarding, and replying to the mail at their terminals.

Access to commercial data bases. The end-user computing industry includes numerous external sources for accessing useful data via dial-up telephone connection using a modem. Companies offering such libraries of data operate much like time-sharing services of the past or the bulletin boards of personal computer user clubs. Access to such commercial data bases is generally available on a fee-for-usage basis. Large publishing companies, for example, frequently provide access to a broad range of data bases, including population demographics and statistics, and bibliographic material in health care and related sciences.

Vendor marketing strategies. Vendor marketing uses this emerging technology directly when marketing presentations are held in a potential customer's office using portable personal computers to demonstrate a software package, or perhaps a subset modified to make the marketing presentation more successful. During a software demonstration on a portable terminal in the customer's office, for example, the modified version might allow presentation of the first few steps of a lengthy data entry sequence, followed by a special command to accelerate the remainder of the sequence. Vendor marketing presentations incorporating this technology are extremely effective because they present the software and hardware products realistically, stimulating the customer's desire to use computer technology to solve his or her record keeping problem.

Marketing targets: Customers within the hospital. A description of the end-user computing industry requires an analysis of potential customers and their reactions to opportunities for using personal computers, as well as cautionary remarks about frequent pitfalls the vulnerable customer may fall into. A prime marketing target for vendors of personal computing technology is the overworked hospital department or the department that has a serious organization and management problem. A polished demonstration creating a report that would seem to solve all the department's problems can be extremely persuasive to an overworked manager. The report's presence on the screen makes personal computer usage seem so tantalizingly easy that the customer may impulsively purchase the software and hardware being demonstrated, totally unaware until after installation of its hidden complexities and difficulties. Only experienced users are aware of key issues such as where the data are to come from, on what timing cycle, how to ensure data quality, and the difficulty of using data elements other than those included in the package. Prospective buyers should have an experienced information systems professional involved in such decisions.

Vendors also frequently aim their marketing at the personal computer user who has risen to the level of departmental expert and who, for personal reasons, wants to work at the technology's leading edge. Such a user is a prime prospect for purchasing the latest high-technology software and hardware. Managers should be aware of who these people are and be aware of vendor marketing influences on them.

Another vulnerable marketing target is the person who is marginally competent in the use of personal computers and who has had minor success. Probably self-taught and confident, though not yet battle-scarred and skeptical, this individual can often be led by vendors to venture beyond his or her actual capability, ignorant not only of the financial risk involved, but also of the risks to the productivity of others in the department as they try to use the new technology. Failure with a new package or system can destroy the credibility of the individual's previous personal computer successes.

The influence of personal computer user clubs. Large personal computer clubs also affect the market in many cities. These clubs usually hold monthly meetings featuring speakers who may be vendor representatives describing their products and future products. Special interest groups within the clubs may meet more frequently to discuss common interests in special areas, such as Lotus 1-2-3, or special applications, such as the use of personal computer technology in the health care industry. The clubs also allow members to purchase products at discounts and to share software libraries.

Personal computer clubs frequently also have electronic bulletin boards that members access over telephone lines using their personal computers and modems. The bulletin boards allow users to obtain news, ask and answer questions of each other in an electronic conferencing forum, and through that same process, contribute and obtain software. The software obtained in this way, sometimes called *shareware,* may be very useful to health care institutions. Unfortunately, it may also be the software most likely to contain the software virus problems described in Chapter 4.

Consultants and free-lance professionals. Consultants and free-lance professionals usually assume leadership roles in computer user clubs and local chapters of professional societies to gain visibility and make contact with potential clients. Consulting opportunities in the use of personal computers are good, and several forces fuel this trend.

First, user departments who want to maintain independence from institutional information services departments would often rather purchase assistance from outside consultants than expose their intents and possible mistakes to the control influences of an internal information services organization. On the other hand, the internal information services organization simply may not have the time to support all user support requests. In another variation, a particular end-user computing project may sound so easy to accomplish that a department believes it can accomplish its objective using much less of the outside consultant's time than is ultimately required.

The competence of consultants or free-lancers varies considerably; therefore, the prospective employing organization will be wise to proceed with caution. Many free-lance entrepreneurs are self-taught and have nothing more than minor and fairly simple successes behind them. They may naively take on institutional tasks for which they have no real qualifications. Furthermore, while free-lancers are usually able to develop systems that they themselves can use, they typically make great mistakes when building systems that include tasks that will be assigned to clerical people who have no computer skills. A system that functions successfully, for example, must have built-in controls that prevent or detect data entry errors. Self-taught free-lancers often know little about, and are even less concerned about, such controls.

Recruiting employees with computer skills. Applicants for personal computer support positions whose skills and experience are limited to those acquired in the earlier days of amateur personal computer use, when the challenge was to operate a fairly simple software package, may prove inadequate for current positions. Shaky credentials cannot equip candidates to move into an environment attempting to build and manage departmental networks accommodating several concurrent users. Minimal skills and successes simply don't provide a platform from which to expect many successes.

This is not to suggest that highly qualified personal computer consultants and free-lance people are not available. Likewise, there are many personal computer support people who really can help build and manage networks. Because the field is so new, however, there is great danger of not being able to distinguish the qualified from the unqualified until it is too late.

Usage Patterns in End-User Computing

The market for personal computer technology is not a single, homogeneous market. Within a health care institution, for example, several different types of usage patterns for this technology exist. First, there is typical usage in a standard office environment. Here, personal computers are used mainly for their word-processing capabilities, possibly incorporating a spreadsheet application for tracking the departmental budget. In addition, they may be used for other administrative activities, such as recording lists of problems or projects and related details such as target dates and status.

A second, more sophisticated group of users, employing different products and skills, is found in a similar but larger office or clinical environment.

This group uses networks to share data files, equipment such as printers, and software, and possibly for sending electronic mail within the network.

The third group of users requires much more complex interconnections with larger computers. These users rely on personal computers as intelligent workstations to combine work processes and data with hospital information systems on larger computers and other personal computers in networks, thereby performing functions not otherwise possible.

Personal computers as independent workstations

Personal computers that are used as traditional independent workstations in many departments throughout a health care institution, for word processing and other simple record keeping, need not be connected to networks. They may be used, for example, to record in-services attended by employees in a department or work unit.[10]

Independent personal computer workstations also may be used to contain an electronic version of departmental reference material. Nursing procedures, for example, may be written and maintained at a central location, but they also can be distributed to each nursing work unit on diskettes, making them available electronically as well as in bound manuals. With such an application, special software allows a user to enter a key word, such as a part of the human anatomy or a special nursing procedure, and thereby initiate a search of all instructions for the presence of that word or phrase. The user can then retrieve, review, and print the instruction that is most relevant to the immediate work issue.

A personal computer used as an independent workstation is also an ideal tool for recording and processing confidential data such as the executive and management payroll. This method affords higher-level salaries and personal data more confidentiality than they would have if included in the normal payroll system.

Interconnected personal computers: Sharing work and data

Personal computers connected into networks that share work and data perform functions similar to those of the minicomputer just a few years ago. Because personal computers are less expensive, more adaptable, and more useful as independent workstations, personal computer networks tend to displace minicomputers for many departmental record-keeping applications. Personal computers interconnected for these applications have the advantage of decentralized computer capacity for maximum productivity and responsiveness to the individual user. They also offer access to centralized resources when necessary.

Health care applications most appropriate for this shared, cooperative processing capability are those sharing data bases that are not too large for this technology's disk drives. A medical staff office, for example, might use a small networked record-keeping system to contain information necessary for the reappointment process and for continuing medical education (CME) record keeping. Clinical departments, such as small labs, can use personal computers instead of minicomputers to gain computing power while also integrating powerful word processing for transcription and other office correspondence. Administrative departments can implement networks that allow several administrative and secretarial people to share files of data. A dietary department can use networked computers to maintain and print information about menus, recipes, and possibly inventory, sharing data among several people and integrating related record keeping such as inventory management and menu planning.

Silent partners: Personal computers and large computers

The most promising and, at the same time, the most difficult and challenging use of personal computers involves operating them in concert with larger computers to perform important HIS information processing requirements. Personal computers on nursing stations, for example, will almost certainly evolve to be capable of performing functions that require data and programs resident on both the nursing station personal computers and larger networked computers, called servers. The user of such a personal computer will be totally unconcerned with, and possibly unaware of, the personal computer's connection with the server computer.

Another possible application is a computer system for tracking work orders in construction and renovation services departments. Work orders for renovation and construction require that all costs of supplies, outside purchases, outside services, and inside services be consolidated and charged to the departments involved, either as operating expenses or as capital expenses, depending on the circumstances. Using traditional methods, construction and renovation charges are compiled from various vendor documents after a project's completion, when labor and other inside expenses are allocated. An internal charge is then made to the department involved— many months after the work is completed and at a time when no management controls or other attention can control the project or its costs. On the other hand, an automated system, combining the technology of large computer business systems with personal computer systems, can streamline this process considerably. Such a system is able to access automatically data available in the work records of the construction and renovation departments, consolidate the data with invoices and purchase orders from the large computers' business systems, print reports of accumulated costs on the small computers, and then automatically integrate consolidated data into the general ledger on the larger computers at month-end.

Interconnected large computers and personal computers might also be useful in processing radiology orders and results. Orders placed through large-computer order entry terminals can be automatically transferred to a network of personal computers that are interconnected to support management of orders and transcription of results, using word-processing software that is integrated into the system. The results can then be automatically sent back to the larger computer. Here, results can be displayed in many ways and at several locations, and they can be accessed from remote locations such as physicians' offices.

Operating room record keeping could also benefit from this client/server technology. Inventory items, physician preference lists, and other record keeping can take place on a network of personal computers, but the operating room scheduling data can be made available to a larger computer by means of a direct computer-to-computer linkage. The system could provide the necessary operating room logs as well as a wide range of reports covering management of the operating rooms, from utilization reports to room turnaround reports.

This type of interconnection may also provide an excellent means for gaining flexible access to comprehensive data bases. Although software packages are available for entering data and using data bases within a personal computer, data may be more easily obtained by automatically linking the personal computer to larger computers that routinely accumulate data bases as part of an operational process. Department heads and head nurses, for instance, could be provided with direct access to monthly financial and statistical data that they would otherwise receive on monthly financial reports. That data, extracted from the larger data base under appropriate security controls, can be analyzed in row and column format, with explanations of variances entered manually and the results printed using a software package such as Lotus 1-2-3. Similarly, staff analysts might access revenue data and associated details involving departments, services, procedures, physicians, and the resulting month-to-month trends.

In addition to the examples described, end-user computing may be readily applied to many types of management analyses. Marketing analyses of market segments, market share, and competition, for example, are handled relatively simply using end-user computing. End-user computing is widely used in health care for financial analyses, planning, and various types of statistical analyses, including productivity.[11]

End-user computing can be used for case-mix analyses and cost-accounting analyses by integrating data from various sources, including patient charge data, departmental procedures, patient data from medical records abstracting files, patient classification or patient acuity data, and clinical data when applicable. Considering the importance of these types of analyses to the health care industry today, the relevance of end-user computing to health care is readily apparent.

Managing End-User Computing

The following sections provide managers guidance in making decisions about use of end-user computing in health care, including when to make use of this technology, what technology to select, and how to monitor the progress of an effort to make use of this technology.

Balancing value against risk of waste and failure

The prospect of end-user computing in health care entails great potential for improved service and increased productivity. At the same time, it also entails a risk of waste and failure as great as the prospect for improved performance. Case histories document modest successes with personal computers at many institutions, yet the serious shortcomings of ambitious projects in numerous hospitals have resulted in considerable skepticism at the promise of widespread, successful personal computer and networking technology. Accordingly, major concerns about the wasteful proliferation and cost justification for this technology have begun to surface.

Identifying and evaluating opportunities

Selections to optimize the personal computer investment. As requirements are defined and acquisition decisions are made, a hospital will want to determine continually that requirements are real and justified and that what is taking place is not technological whim or experimentation masquerading as improvement. Novice users, for example, sometimes expect technology to solve problems actually caused by poor organization of work in a department and may seek automated solutions that are neither valuable nor practicable. In a similar manner, power users at the other end of the spectrum, and at the leading edge of PC technology, may be motivated to press for innovation merely for its experimental value. Even careful experienced users may make mistakes based on false confidence from minor successes, and reach beyond their proficiency for solutions that are not feasible, since the newest automation proposals almost invariably prove more difficult and risky than previous, simpler attempts. Bolstered by intense vendor marketing, these practices can lead to waste of hospital resources and major problems in optimal use of this promising new technology.[12] Although the wasted investment in any given department may be modest, the potential for similar failures in many departments poses a much greater risk that could exist undetected without adequate management controls over proliferation of this technology.

Approval controls. To reduce the risk of investing in frivolous or ill-defined projects, approval should be granted only for projects that relate to specific objectives. A hospital manager should ensure that requirements are always defined by knowledgeable users thoroughly familiar with the actual systems or enhancements being installed, and that requests for purchases are documented with substantial evidence of need.

Periodic reviews, especially for those projects that are pressing the leading edge of technology or that directly or indirectly involve large expenditures, serve as further controls against wasteful investment of hospital resources. Such a review process, moreover, allows the hospital's managers to learn from mistakes made, and possibly avoid those same mistakes and problems in subsequent projects.

Recording acquisitions. Regardless of a technology's potential benefits, one absolute requirement is that purchases of personal computer technology be recorded. The location of each personal computer and its general purpose or objective, along with information on the model numbers, main user, and major purpose, should be recorded. Without such documentation, no method exists for later evaluating whether or not the project is successful and, therefore, should be extended with later support.[13,14]

Guidance and support for technology selection and learning

Centralized support to provide advice and problem solving. The expertise of the information services organization can be used to prevent failures of end-user computing projects and waste of institutional resources on such efforts.[15] A common organizational pattern calls for a specialized support center that provides expertise and assistance to users and potential users of end-user computing. With such an arrangement, potential new users may be invited to visit a central location where they can see and experiment with and watch demonstrations of new technology. The temporary loan of computer equipment to potential users also allows personnel some time to understand new technology before purchasing it.

This type of centralized support function is sometimes called an *information center,* a name used throughout the information technology industry to identify a special group of support people and their work location.[16] The information center is usually located in an office area that users can visit to obtain support and guidance.

The center frequently is also a first line of support for problem-solving assistance. This support function includes routine record keeping about the nature of problems, which in turn enables management to draw conclusions about the quality of products in use and any need for additional training.

In addition to the above functions, the center is often the focus of training, offering instruction on some topics directly, and periodically arranging for outside experts to provide training on special subjects. An information center can also provide a means for communication among users that employ similar end-user computing technology. Periodic newsletters, user surveys, open houses, and show-and-tell meetings are useful for this purpose. Through this process, a group can multiply potential benefits throughout an institution, raising users' awareness of how others are applying technology.

Standardization for efficient learning and support. A centralized support center can also evaluate vendor products and urge the use of fairly standardized equipment and software, which allows the institution to benefit from the efficiencies associated with many departments using similar technology. In the interest of work sharing, data sharing, transferring skills from department to department, and generally improving the learning curve of experience within an institution, some limits on the diversity of products should be encouraged.

Developing solutions for users. Information center support personnel serve a twofold purpose when they develop computer programs and devise solutions for users. First, they facilitate the project's positive contribution to the user department. As a by-product, they offer the users a solid first experience and possibly a sample of computer software that they can clone for future use. From that point, users' expertise will evolve at an individualized pace.

Guidance on data availability, accuracy, controls, and security. Users should also be guided on such issues as protection of data against fraud, data confidentiality, and other control issues.[17] Guidance should also be provided on the availability of data, its accuracy, and its cycle of availability. As a result, end-user access to widely distributed data bases can be channeled and monitored.

To provide such guidance, a member of the information services support staff should identify the corporate data bases residing in each computer, the processes by which data are collected, the conditions necessary for data accuracy, and the timing relationships between or among data. For example, data, left vaguely undefined in islands of personal computer use, could be misleading if its collection and analytical cycle is out of phase with other important information flow, as in periodically reported financial information. Or the data may be redundantly or inconsistently processed from month to month, so that its credibility erodes. The challenge is to identify all distributed data bases that are important to the hospital's mainstream information cycles and then to define and communicate these details, data element by data element, to all users who could potentially need to use the data.

Reviews of value: Monitoring after approval

Periodic evaluations at project milestones. End-user computing systems are intended to benefit, not burden, users, generating identifiable payoffs to the departments involved. Therefore, in addition to functioning correctly, they must operate smoothly and dependably, without requiring daily problem solving or other corrective intervention. To ensure that projects incorporating computer technology are generating optimal benefits to the institution, managers should periodically evaluate all projects at clearly defined milestones, such as the completion of installation of equipment, the completion of the first prototype version of the system, and the completion of the first phase of training. The objective of such evaluations is not necessarily to eliminate projects, but to justify providing end-user computing capabilities to as many work groups and employees as possible throughout the health care institution. At the same time, managers must prevent the haphazard spread and wasted effort of uninformed use by providing continuous guidance in the selection of application projects. In the absence of such management control, unorganized use of computers causes not only waste of valuable resources, but also loss of confidence in the technology.

Implementing the hybrid technology of end-user computing is a challenge beyond anything we have ever faced in the general management of our hospitals. End-user computing, however, will become increasingly fundamental to hospital success; therefore, management must invest the continuing attention necessary for fully capitalizing on its promise.

Creeping commitments. Inevitably, mistakes will occur and problems will arise; in such instances, users and middle managers may be tempted to resort to increasingly greater investments aimed at solving problems, camouflaging failures, or merely gaining more time. For example, a user in an administrative or clinical department may acquire a personal computer and related equipment and software, invest a great deal of hospital resources in early usage, then determine that it cannot be used effectively unless it is interconnected with another computer in another department, which requires greater investment for additional equipment and software. Similarly, personal computer users who are involved in less-than-successful PC projects may try to use their failures to justify even greater investments and more complex technology. They may seek interconnection and complex integration with other technology to help bail themselves out or to camouflage their failures and gain more time. Such cycles can continue indefinitely, with additional purchases made and more and more hospital resources invested, without realizing the expected benefits. Creeping commitments are easy to fall into; the best insurance against them is management's consistent analysis of problems and mistakes and wariness of investment of add-on technology unless it has been rigorously determined to be of real value to the hospital.

Monitoring the work of obsessed personal computer users. Occasionally personal computer users may become intrigued with the magic of computer technology, dedicating more and more time to exploring the possibilities of the computers on their desks, and often becoming almost indifferent to their actual job responsibilities. In such cases, productivity may decrease substantially. Furthermore, these computer enthusiasts may influence their managers to purchase the latest fads in hardware or software so that they can spend time tinkering with the technology. Unmonitored and without effective management restraint, such personnel can lead their departments, and possibly other departments, down inappropriate paths—sacrificing hospital resources to their own preoccupation with personal computer technology.

Assessing the influence of vendor marketing. Vendor marketing is also a powerful force that can counter efforts to evaluate and control expenditures. Vendors who exaggerate a technology's benefits and downplay the effort and expense required for its successful use are another cause of projects that fail to meet expectations. A user's first experiences with personal computers are often deceptively easy. Such a user, buoyed by preliminary success, is often particularly susceptible to a skillfully staged marketing demonstration and may be persuaded to buy another product that he or she will not be able to use successfully without considerable support by others. Potential users are all too frequently led to the false conclusion that personal computer concepts and skills can be mastered easily and that users can, with little outside guidance, design and implement comprehensive systems. When hospitals closely monitor these projects, vendors who are guilty of such practices will be identified and possibly excluded from further business with the hospital, and users who fall victim to such practices will be identified and be subjected to even closer monitoring.

Supporting successful projects with follow-on approvals. A monitoring and approval process can be a powerful means of communicating support for successful projects and of establishing and reinforcing appropriate criteria for selecting end-user computing opportunities, especially when a variety of alternatives exist that may not be in the hospital's best interests. Different departments and individuals are constantly moving through different stages of proficiency with the technology, and the deliberate dissemination of details about successes and failures communicates to them, as well as to management, the ingredients required for a successful project. An evaluation and approval process is an invaluable tool for refining end-user computing efforts within a hospital.

Potential for Additional Benefits in the Future

End-user computer technology holds great potential for health care applications. It is becoming, and will continue to be, a fundamental part of hospitals' information systems.

Ease of use

Increasing ease of use, anticipated in the near future, will maximize end-user computing's potential. Further advancements in the technology will provide much greater processing power and storage capacity than was imagined a few years ago. These capabilities will lead to an abundance of new and useful applications in health care.

There has been little vendor incentive thus far, however, to provide common conventions in the use of keyboards and screen pointing devices and in the appearance of video screens. Use of the many different application software packages, therefore, demand more learning and skills than would be required if common conventions existed among them. Moreover, inconsistencies among software packages lead to reduced user proficiency, higher error rates, and reduced performance speed. Users have become frustrated with these inconsistencies, and in reaction, larger vendors in the industry are beginning to show an interest in moving toward establishing some standard. To achieve standardization, however, we will have to start over with many products, reinventing some of their major parts, and standardizing video screen formats and usage conventions. Driving forces in this area are very powerful, and we can expect continued heavy market turmoil to continue for years. Life cycles of most products during this period will last no more than about three years.

Growing desktop power as a driving force for more automation

The fast-paced growth of end-user computing technology is itself becoming a force driving us to enhance already successful systems and to automate more processes in departments where successful projects have given credibility to the technology. Clearly, successful use and the briskly evolving technology are powerful factors leading us to implement this technology in ever more complex and critical processes within our hospitals.

Graphics enhancements. In particular, recent advancements in computer graphics hardware and software are providing new output options for end-user computing. High-resolution and color graphic printers, plotters, and advanced video displays are providing a palette of output options that will enable users to display textual, numeric, and graphical image data in a wide variety of graphic formats. For example, advancements will allow diagnostic images to be presented on video screens that will also contain text and numerical data. Digitized copies of special forms, and even handwritten notes, may be displayed on such high-resolution graphic devices in the future.

Larger files of data. As desktop workstations become more powerful, use of spreadsheet products like Lotus 1-2-3 will be stretched to handle larger and larger files of data. When first introduced, these spreadsheet products were used to process fairly straightforward files of rows and columns of data. But, over several years of enthusiastic use, applications have naturally grown to include far larger sets of data as innovative users have pressed them to process data bases far beyond the accounting worksheets for which the software packages were initially designed. Large sets of operating room case statistics, for example, may be consolidated from statistics collected over a long period of time. Or, using networking interconnections, data may be consolidated from several sources, such as large sets of statistics from several operating rooms. In particular, using an interconnection with a mainframe computer, data may be downloaded from large data bases. The data capacity requirements of end-user computing have slowly grown substantially, and as a result, the market will be pressured to deliver workstations with greater and greater capability for handling large volumes of data.

Integrating end-user computing into mainstream information processing

Broader data access. A major concern among future users of end-user computing will be the increased capability to locate, gain access to, and process data from a hospital's operational transactions. For example, the complexity and comprehensiveness of management analyses are requiring that data be derived and consolidated from two or more separate data sources within an institution.[18] To provide this capability in the future, enhanced networks and interconnections among computers will provide shared data gathering and data usage. User-friendly methods of sharing data and work across the networks will become available.

Data are an important hospital resource. To use data effectively we must identify the data bases distributed throughout the hospital's computers; define the data elements, their data collection cycles, and other important characteristics; and structure them into the information processing cycles of the hospital. Chapter 8 includes an in-depth discussion of the quality and integrity of data available in these independent processes.

Changing the conceptual model. We must shift our thinking about the function of end-user computing. We began by describing it as a process through which users independently use computer technology and selected corporate data to do their work. As such, it was an independent process, incidental to a hospital's mainstream information processing. In the future, however, we must begin to think of end-user computing as part of the mainstream, not simply as islands of independent use. In a health care institution, clinicians will want to make use of broad and comprehensive patient data. To make those data available, computer systems throughout the institution must be integrated into the hospital's mainstream information flow. These management opportunities and advances in end-user computing will drive us toward more and more data sharing and integrated work.

Notes

1. J. F. Rockart and C. V. Bullen, eds., *The Rise of Managerial Computing* (Homewood, IL: Dow Jones–Irwin, 1986), pp. xii, 376.
2. Ibid., p. xiii.
3. Ibid., p. 314.
4. Ibid., p. 313.
5. Ibid., p. 311.
6. W. P. Pierskalla and D. Woods, "Computers in Hospital Management and Improvements in Patient Care—New Trends in the United States," *Journal of Medical Systems* 12, no. 6 (1988): 412.
7. Ibid.
8. D. H. McConnell and M. A. Brenner, "HIS: The Clinician's Role," *Computers in Healthcare* (June 1989): 20–22, 24.
9. T. A. Pryor, "Computerized Nurse Charting," *International Journal of Clinical Monitoring and Computing* (1989): 178.

10. B. F. Minard, "PC Workstations: Vital Link in a Distributed Information System," *Proceedings of the 1988 Annual Health Care Systems Conference* (Chicago: Healthcare Information and Management Systems Society, American Hospital Association, 1987), pp. 99–104.

11. Rockart and Bullen, *The Rise of Managerial Computing,* p. 314.

12. F. G. Withington, "Coping with Computer Proliferation," *Harvard Business Review* 58, no. 3 (May–June 1980): 152–64.

13. B. F. Minard, "Effective Information Systems Planning," *Computers in Healthcare* (July 1987): 40–49.

14. B. F. Minard, "Managing the Hospital's Portfolio of Information Systems," *Healthcare Strategic Management* 5, no. 1 (1987): 16–22.

15. Rockart and Bullen, *The Rise of Managerial Computing,* pp. 307–8.

16. Ibid., p. 313.

17. Withington, "Coping with Computer Proliferation," pp. 152–64.

18. Rockart and Bullen, *The Rise of Managerial Computing,* p. 295.

6

INFORMATION SYSTEMS SELECTION
AND ACQUISITION

Once a health care institution's steering committee decides to acquire an essential computer information system, speedy and efficient acquisition and implementation of the system become critical factors in the institution's success. The complex process of selecting project team participants, assigning responsibilities, assessing current systems and procedures, defining new requirements, analyzing alternative acquisition opportunities, selecting a system, negotiating contracts, and successfully implementing the chosen system requires expert management of a dedicated team of employees from diverse departments.

For example, every processing capability must be carefully defined. Bewildering alternatives must be scrutinized before making decisions.[1] And, ultimately, the institution's success or failure could depend on timely and effective acquisition and implementation. Success can give the institution a competitive edge in its market, while extended delays and the system's failure to perform as expected may instead prompt a devastating cycle of management problems. This chapter focuses on system selection and acquisition. System implementation processes are described in Chapter 7.

The Information Systems Marketplace:
History and Complexity

The earliest computer information systems simply automated existing routine work; consequently, complex system acquisition decisions were not important executive management issues. In that era, hardware was acquired, and software was either free or developed by computer programming professionals employed by the institutions preparing to use the systems.

As technology advanced, expectations rose. Myriad sophisticated software projects were undertaken—and many of them failed. Today's marketplace and methods grew out of those early failures and unfulfilled expectations.

Seeds of Today's Problems and Opportunities

Computer processes in the earliest business information systems were relatively easy to define, and the resulting computerized capability usually met expectations. For example, an accountant and a computer programmer worked together to specify how a computer system would duplicate a portion of a manual accounting or clerical process. These same two individuals then installed, tested, and implemented that system.

Computer vendors sold hardware in those early days, but no software vendors existed. To help sell hardware, vendors promoted formation of user groups that shared and exchanged software among institutions. Hardware vendors also developed and otherwise obtained general purpose and business software that they made available to customers free or at low cost. For example, IBM provided hospitals with the patient accounting software known as SHAS (Shared Hospital Accounting System).

In that early era, institutions employed programming staffs that were fairly successful in developing information systems from free and low-cost software, using computer languages and other software development tools, such as report writers. Early software systems were called *batch processing systems* because they processed batches of data: batches of accounts payable invoices, batches of payroll time cards, batches of patient charges, and batches of printed checks. These programs relied on simple logic, systematically processing each data element in each record of each batch while checking for predefined validity conditions. The logic of the work flow was easy for users to define, the resulting computer programming was not too complex, programming errors were easily detected, and periodic computer processing failures were relatively easy to recover and restart.

Eventually, capability for on-line systems emerged to displace purely batch systems. On-line systems offered direct user interaction from terminals in user work areas, such as in the patient registration department, thus permitting transfer of the data entry work closer to the user's point of work. Such systems were especially valuable if data required frequent updating and the data entry results had to be immediately available to others using the system, as in patient registration systems that were known originally as ADT systems, since they were used to enter the admissions, discharges, and transfers of patients. As on-line systems grew in number and usefulness, the complexity and comprehensiveness of systems increased. Increased levels of both computer programming difficulty and demands for planning and managing computer systems, however, were not fully acknowledged at the time. As a result, most early on-line systems did not serve their hospitals well. The systems' marginal capabilities and frequent failures made them less useful than expected.

In addition, users were unprepared for the skills they needed to operate the new on-line systems—and for the issues of work management that consequently arose. For example, users' declarations about the logical flow of their work were often poorly defined, and many reprogramming efforts were typically required to gradually transform the programmed work flow into a useable form. The resulting need to continually change computer programs made the work of computer programming much more difficult and time consuming, and programming problems occurred frequently.

The underlying software of the relatively primitive operating systems and telecommunications systems was itself flawed and the source of many problems. As a result, computer processing problems could have several different causes, and consequently, the potential combinations of causes made problem diagnosis and problem solving extremely difficult. Furthermore, occasional problems in recovery and restart from such complex problems caused additional problems.

For these reasons, the era of complex on-line systems led to major failures of computer systems projects in health care as well as in other industries. Project activity fell well behind schedules, costs grew to multiples of budgeted amounts, and the systems often failed when placed in operation. Moreover, managers sometimes caused failures by overestimating the technology's capability, overestimating their ability to successfully define processes chosen for automation, and underestimating the effort ultimately required to complete projects successfully. Frequently, consultants were engaged to analyze failures and propose remedies. Unfortunately, the analyses often generated overwhelmingly detailed staff work and incredibly high costs, strained working relationships, and prescribed detailed plans for restarting the project, often under the consultants' management. Frequently, these remedial efforts also subsequently failed.

Eventually, good intentions and wisdom gleaned from failure did lead to successes. These successes were based on improved ability both to organize and manage projects and to control the work of specifying processes to be automated. This control applied primarily to the precise definition of system specifications, since researchers of that era determined that institutions "will be more successful in translating management goals into working systems the more specifically the goals are defined."[2] Successes resulted also from effective, well-defined methods of selecting among alternatives and from the more effective and cooperative work of groups of people from diverse departments seeking together to define and select the system's major characteristics. For example, researchers found that "mixed teams are more likely to be successful in MIS [management information system] projects."[3] Furthermore, they discovered that good management of these work groups adds quality to ideas, clarity to the precise statement of problems and objectives, and focus to the quality of the group's resulting work.[4] These collective ingredients of success formed a firm foundation on which today's models for management of computer system acquisition projects could grow.

The emergence of packaged software also offered solutions to several early problems. First, packaged software capabilities essentially defined how certain standardized work processes must be organized in order to make use of the software, relieving each institution of the need to specify work procedures in painstaking detail. In a conventional process of paying vendor invoices, for example, an accounts payable software package would provide standard procedures for the accounts payable department. Instead of trying to define how their departmental work should be performed, users accepted the automated standard procedures and changed their work procedures to match those of the package. Second, because the software package's predefined work flow eliminated much of the difficult work of defining detailed work flow, it also reduced the risk of problems caused by flawed declarations of the precise procedures required. Third, installed software produced fewer operational computer problems. Because the software was already in use somewhere else, many programming errors had already been located and corrected. Consequently, the market for software packages grew dramatically during this period.

Although the market provided software that performed defined functions, such as accounts payable functions, institutions still had to deal with the passing of data among systems, called the *interface* among systems, such as that between an accounts payable system and a general ledger system. These interfaces are the means by which data are automatically transferred among the systems, as, for example, accounts payable data are transferred to a general ledger system so that expenses may be included in monthly departmental reports. These complex interfaces were the source of many problems that weakened the value of purchased software packages. As a result, vendors realized the market value of offering a broader product line of several interconnected software packages, streamlining these interfaces under a single design influence. Seizing this opportunity, vendors acquired other vendors and rights to others' software, filling out their product lines and gaining greater marketing prospects by offering more integrated solutions and the capability to reduce interface problems among systems. For a customer, however, there was potential disadvantage in selecting a combination of systems from one vendor: no single vendor offered a combination of systems that was as good as its—and other vendors'—best individual system.

But vendors continued to improve their integrated combinations of computer systems, adding greater capability and greater complexity. This ongoing effort to integrate systems is one force causing the partial consolidation of computer markets, a trend recently also driven by the emerging networking technology described in Chapter 4. Newer, more integrated products facilitate file sharing and work sharing among computers. They also potentially provide user work functions at a single workstation, regardless of the location of several possible interconnected computers that perform the computer processing.

The resulting new system capabilities are more useful to institutions and will likely be easier for users. But this new stage in the evolution of computer systems is also creating far more complex systems, making the importance of carefully managing the systems acquisition process more crucial than ever before.

Complex Interdependencies

Despite—and, to a certain extent, because of—the great capability and many available options offered by comprehensive integrated software packages, complex system interdependencies plague the system acquisition process. Even after a system is acquired and implemented, complex interdependencies could lead to poor system performance or even failure. These complex interdependencies exist among installed computer systems and planned computer systems, among each system's processing functions and data elements, and among interconnected software and hardware products that operate together and depend on each other to successfully provide desired system capability. These many interdependencies must be thoroughly analyzed, understood, and planned for if a system is to be successful.

The processing interdependencies of an institution's comprehensive information systems are highly complex. Many complex processing functions depend upon each other and on data elements—and both of these, in turn, depend on methods of input and output. For example, the work processes and data elements that are required to allow entry and updating of patient demographic details, such as age or illness, are usually part of a hospital's patient registration process, but the accuracy of the processing of a computerized pharmacy system depends on those same data elements. The data elements and processing functions of the information system's many parts must be integrated into the complex work flow of many other of the institution's manual processes and information systems, so that the institution's information systems function as a single, coordinated system. Research has shown that the more successful this integration, the greater the likelihood of the information system's success.[5]

Interdependencies also exist among groups of people who together perform the work of an institution. And as the cooperative clinical work of these people is changed by the waves of new technology, differing group perspectives add complexity to the system acquisition process. For example, order and results management systems organize the work of physicians, nursing personnel, and ancillary department personnel. However, these different groups view their responsibilities toward a patient differently, requiring that a system address the concerns of all the groups. Nurses face voluminous information documentation during continuous, round-the-clock attention to the patient, while physicians have a more periodic and compartmentalized view of information about patient status. The work of ancillary department personnel, on the other hand, is driven by information on work lists, information that is created by others who are closer to the patient.

Consequently, although the ready availability of packaged software once lessened requirements to define work processes in great detail, the complexity of interconnected and integrated information systems has partially neutralized that advantage. As part of the system acquisition process, the project team must once again give great attention to the task of analyzing, understanding, and defining the institution's complex work processes in great detail. Success is usually achieved by requiring that the project team begin the selection and acquisition process by conducting a thorough step-by-step analysis and definition of the necessary data elements, processing functions, and their relationships with one another.[6-8]

Other Major Complexities and Vulnerabilities

Unfortunately, the system acquisition process poses a threat to executive management's control over planning and prioritizing the acquisition of computer systems. The process exposes the institution both to vendors' strong, influential marketing and to employees' unpredictable response to this influence. During the acquisition process, assigned participants make critical decisions about whether a given computer processing function is justified and will improve operations, or is an unjustified overhead that will simply waste the institution's resources. As a result, the institution risks possible acquisition of a product other than what was planned and assigned priority by the executive-level steering committee. For example, a vendor may subtly sell a major add-on product, divert attention from flaws in its products, or convince project team participants to pursue tangents or special interests in which the vendor specializes.

The institution is also vulnerable to traditional and historical problems of underestimated costs, work efforts, and project durations. Just as was frequently the case in the past, the inexperience of managers and staff can lead to failure. Even without vendors' strong marketing influence, extensions and commitments naturally proliferate after the project starts. On top of these creeping commitments to broaden the project's scope, the task of estimating the amount and duration of computer systems related work is very difficult. There is simply no accurate way to predict and measure all the work of the many people who must contribute to the effort.

During the acquisition process, project teams must also be concerned about the threat of obsolescence because new systems may become available during the time frame of the planned system acquisition. This vulnerability is even greater in large and complex institutions, where the acquisition and implementation process requires a fairly long time period. Here, there is a risk that the obsolescence could even overlap the acquisition and implementation process. And vulnerability to obsolescence in a large and complex institution is a double-edged sword. The process of later replacement may also be more difficult, because more functions will be automated and in use by more staff members at that time, making future conversion to a new system more extensive and difficult.

These not insubstantial vulnerabilities become even more critical as technological complexity and risk of failure increase. During the system acquisition process, assigned employees make critical and complex decisions affecting the fit of the system to the culture and structure of the institution, and they establish the foundation for several years of successful or unsuccessful system usage. With all these opportunities to fail, the future success of an institution could actually hinge on the effectiveness of the system acquisition process.

Sources of Systems

Powerful market forces are causing great volatility in both the health care software and computer hardware markets. Market forces, such as health care cost pressures, changed expectations of users, changes in the market position and strategy of hardware and software vendors, and advancing technology itself, resulted in dramatic changes in the health care information systems markets during 1988 and 1989, as many vendor changes occurred. Vendors formed alliances with each other, created joint ventures, merged, were spun off, and sometimes disappeared altogether.

Hardware vendors

Some manufacturers market computers on which the software of application software vendors operates, while some provide extensive portfolios of software and gain considerable revenue by marketing a variety of their own software products. Their objective in marketing a combination of software and hardware is to provide a single marketing contact point, providing control and added marketing focus for the vendor, while offering convenience for the customer. Their software marketing efforts are also driven by a long-term effect: users' acquisition of additional software ultimately creates a future need to acquire additional hardware.

Hardware vendors that provide both hardware and software potentially offer customers another subtle advantage. Their marketing strategies and plans for software are usually more sensitive to the effects of fast-paced and dramatic upgrades in the underlying technology of hardware and operating system software. These vendors' upgrades to the underlying hardware and operating system software are usually planned several years in advance of their availability to the market. Therefore, hardware manufacturers' compatible software products are more likely to be planned to exploit this changing hardware technology.

For example, major changes in both microcomputer and larger computer hardware have recently occurred every two or three years. Because customers expect software products to be useful for longer than two or three years, any given software package should be expected to operate across the transition of major changes in the underlying hardware technology. As new hardware becomes available, it usually makes new software capability possible—but the old software should also be capable of operating on the new hardware together with the new software.

These dramatic transitions in hardware technology present a special problem for vendors that have large installed customer bases. Hardware vendors are especially aware that they must provide their customers continued compatibility among the continuous stream of their products upgrades; otherwise, current customers would face significant discontinuities in usage in order to make use of new software or hardware technologies of that vendor. If future versions of a vendor's products were not compatible with older versions, customers may see no benefit in staying with the same vendor and may instead select a new hardware vendor. Consequently, hardware vendors are unlikely to market products that do not feature this compatibility, called *upward compatibility*. Purely software vendors, on the other hand, may not have a strategic commitment to such a goal.

Some hardware vendors, however, market little or no software for the health care marketplace, but depend for sales of their hardware on marketing alliances, such as value added remarketing (VAR) agreements with major software firms.

Application software vendors

There are two major advantages to acquiring software instead of designing and developing software systems using a computer programming staff. First, the software is usually already functioning elsewhere. Second, the total cost and implementation period are usually more predictable. On the other hand, the drawback to this strategy is that the hospital is highly dependent on, and to some extent controlled by, the vendor. The hospital is dependent on the quality and responsiveness of the vendor's support staff. And the vendor, by virtue of its commitment (or lack of commitment) to planning, investment, and management of its products' continued evolution, controls the hospital's future capability to enhance its installed software and, therefore, its operating procedures. Moreover, because the hospital is dependent on the vendor, the hospital might fall victim to the vendor's misfortunes in the market: the vendor may encounter cash problems and lose staff, or fail to invest in and improve its products. And the hospital is also subject to whatever pricing strategies the vendor imposes for both future support and future versions of its products.

The growing software market has produced many large firms that develop and market software. Available products range from software for broad corporate purposes, such as general ledgers, to software for major portions of hospital information systems, such as patient accounting, billing, accounts receivable, and clinical systems. Hundreds of application software vendors market software to health care institutions.

Other acquisition possibilities

In another type of acquisition, the hospital customer simply contracts with a vendor to provide the required capability. In one type of such a contract, a hospital simply contracts for shared use of a computer system that is on the vendor's premises, in which case computer terminals are installed on the hospital's premises to connect to the vendor's computer system over telephone lines. In another type of contract, a facilities management contract, the vendor agrees to install, operate, and manage the system on the customer's premises. Several variations of these types of contracts are possible.[9]

Customized computer programming

Despite the spectrum of available vendor support, some customized computer programming is sometimes necessary by either the vendor, the health care institution, or a third party under contract. Software packages support only standard and well-defined work processes and sometimes require considerable computer programming work at the points of interface among software packages. System interfaces usually are customized and tailored to institutions' specially defined requirements, such as different methods for passing data details among patient accounting, general ledger, bank reconciliation, cost accounting, and purchasing and inventory systems. Special customized programming is usually necessary for this tailoring, as well as customized programming for special modifications that are beyond the capabilities provided by software packages.

In some few cases, developing application software by customized computer programming (usually called *in-house computer programming*) is a better alternative than seeking a software package from a vendor. For example, specialized health care institutions like long-term rehabilitation care facilities may require certain unique patient scheduling functions that are not available in the software marketplace. Furthermore, customized computer programming by the health care institution's computer programming staff is probably the best choice if computerization is necessary to meet an institution's specific strategic objective, such as, for example, establishing computerized links between hospital computer systems and physicians' office computer systems. In such a case, the hospital may want to have complete control over the software and not want to allow a newly conceived software capability to be available to competitors.

Selected computer programming is also sometimes justified to customize vendor software products when none can provide a good fit to the hospital's requirements. This situation occurred frequently in the earlier eras of computer usage, and unfortunately the problem continues to exist when vendors define software products without seeking proper guidance from potential customers.

Special software tools

Other special software tools available in the marketplace perform a variety of functions. Some directly enhance processing capability; others aid in system testing and implementation. Still others provide diagnostic and management assistance to customer management personnel responsible for operating and maintaining the acquired systems.

Data base management software, especially supporting relational data bases, is available from several vendors, differing in efficiency, speed of operation, and capability. In addition, several vendors offer report writer software and special inquiry languages. Some of these products qualify as *fourth generation languages* (4GL), which emphasize special advanced features and ease of use by users who are not computer programming professionals. Software to provide networking capability to interconnect computers is also available.

Prototyping software enhances the system implementation process by permitting easy and quick presentation of sample display screens and report formats. This kind of software allows personnel who will ultimately use the system to test and experience the options, and suggest changes before display screen and report details are finalized.

Software is also available to help locate and eliminate errors from software. Some products analyze the logic of computer programs, expertly searching for subtle logic errors that would otherwise be revealed only by system failures. Other available software closely monitors processing under way, scrutinizing functions and diagnosing problems. And available software can monitor and help manage changes to computer program libraries.

Software tools can also provide diagnostic assistance to management personnel who are responsible for operating and maintaining production systems. These tools feature performance indicators such as counts of computer transactions, tabulation and statistical analysis of computer response times, and utilization of data storage space in disk storage units. Other software tools are geared for other computer production management purposes: copying data files to provide backup copies, providing audit trails of computer transactions, automatically scheduling computer processing, and ensuring data security. Still other software performs problem diagnostic activities, such as automatically analyzing network functions and sensing and alerting management of marginal operation even before failures occur.

Where to Find Information, Advice, and Other Assistance

Consultants and other experts

Consultants can provide valuable assistance at many points in a system acquisition project. For example, they may be called upon at the beginning of a project to foster good start-up activities, at major milestones to provide needed technical or managerial expertise, or at a time of crisis to help correct problems or system failures.

Consultants may be used very successfully at the beginning of a project, both to help organize the team and to get the work under way. On the other hand, consultants are occasionally engaged as agents to impose an opinion held by a small group on others. Such a strategy can exert a negative influence on the project.

Consultants may also be engaged to help at selected milestones while a system acquisition project is under way. They can review outcomes of the project's major phases, ensure thoroughness by checking documented system requirements, search for flaws in the system selection process, evaluate and recommend changes to contracts, help negotiate contracts, or pinpoint the causes of dissatisfaction with progress or performance. In these cases, consultants provide expertise and a base of experience that the institution's employees do not have. For example, consultants with special expertise, such as in system integration, may be engaged to evaluate and plan interconnections among systems.

Choosing the right consultant is crucial. Large consulting firms that are part of, or affiliated with, the large accounting firms can handle a project of almost any scope, but are usually very expensive and may not assign personnel with appropriate experience in health care. Some consulting firms specialize in health care information systems and would likely provide competent personnel. Some firms may be able to provide expertise in special niches of health care computing, such as in claims processing, outpatient scheduling, or data security. Academic consultants' expertise is usually specialized based on research interest, such as in expert systems, and their academic schedules frequently preclude commitment to a major, long-term project.

As one final caveat, remember that consultants are business people who are ultimately motivated by profit. They may make recommendations that benefit themselves as much or more than the customer. In particular, carefully evaluate a consultant's recommendations that require the consulting firm's products or the consultant's continued engagement.

Interinstitutional user groups

Interinstitutional user groups are frequently formed by groups of institutions that use the products of a single information systems vendor. These groups provide a valuable forum for sharing information, and they typically have officers, periodic conferences, and advisory councils that guide the evolution of vendor products. One example of a large user group is Health Quest's health care information systems products user group. Called IMPACT, this user group conducts two meetings each year that feature member presentations.

During a system acquisition process, it may be useful to contact members of user groups to gain information about vendor products and vendor relationships. The agenda of recent user group conferences might also offer evidence of system features that have attracted special interest because they are new, changing, or problematic.

When a user group does have an advisory council that prioritizes customers' requests for product changes, these lists of requests, and the prioritized results, can help prospective customers anticipate and assess future versions of vendors' products. User groups may also provide valuable information about useful modifications that customers have made to vendor products. Individual members of user groups may even make some of those modifications available to others.

Professional societies and other industry groups

Professional societies and health care industry groups are also excellent sources of assistance during a system acquisition project. Professional societies, such as the Health Care Information and Management Systems Society (HIMSS), hold annual conferences and publish periodicals that help in understanding, evaluating, and selecting information systems. Health care industry groups, such as the Texas Hospital Association, also provide conferences, periodicals, books, and special committees that focus on issues of special interest during system acquisition projects.

Special standard-setting groups may also provide important assistance. For example, vendors and customers of health care information systems products have formed special committees, such as Health Level 7 (HL-7), that plan standards for exchanging data among computer systems. A vendor's membership on such a committee, and evidence of its conformance with such standards, may be useful information to consider during a system acquisition process.

The Importance of the System Acquisition Process

Planning, discussed in Chapter 2, provides the strategic decisions about systems that should be approved and funded. Under the planning guidelines, executive management controls the priorities, decides which systems should be funded for acquisition, and then approves the projects and assigns project teams to define the systems in greater detail, leading to acquisition and, finally, implementation.

The acquisition process is crucial, and it must be managed well. Successes result from imposing a consistent process for selecting new and enhanced information systems—and assuring that the process is understood by employees, medical staff, management, executives, and board.[10-17] Although interdependencies among institutional processes are many and complex, as are interdependencies among the work of project team members and other hospital management and staff employees, such a process can be successful if it engages broad participation in project teams and is managed by a senior manager or executive who is qualified to manage a project of this complexity.

Managing the Acquisition Process

Compentent Management of Project Teams

Mixed teams from diverse departments

Researchers, including many in health care, have concluded that system acquisition projects (and system implementation projects) are more likely to be successful if they are guided by the cooperative work of balanced teams of employees from diverse departments.[18-24] These project teams include managers, physicians, nurses, and other employees who know the institution's operations and goals well and who understand the complexities of service interactions among departments. Participants are required to analyze details of the institution's procedures, problems, and objectives, and they must be able to translate that information into definitions of requirements.

Inclusion of clinical personnel

Physicians and nurses play a vital role in project teams charged with defining and implementing hospitalwide computer systems. Health care institutions that have included clinical personnel into their information system selection and acquisition processes report that their participation helps to integrate and balance the objectives of patient management, costs management, and quality enhancement in their institutions.[25]

Physicians should be included in the selection process so that the selected system will be one that they can and will use. In many hospitals that have installed information systems that physicians could use, most physicians do not use them, in part because their participation was not sought and obtained, and consequently they were not part of the selection process.[26] Participating physicians should be given important responsibilities for defining system capabilities that will be feasible and useful to them, so that they conclude that the project team is making a good selection, and they will then communicate that conclusion to other physicians. Consequently, physicians will then be more likely to rely on and use the system than would be the case if they did not participate in its selection.[27]

To gain the cooperation of physicians, influential physicians should be identified and consulted.[28] They, or their choice of other physicians, should be included as members of the overall project team or an important work group that is responsible for the system's clinical capabilities.

Project management and leadership

A well-balanced project team requires competent leadership; subcommittees or work groups with assigned responsibilities; a work plan and well-defined task assignments; a method of tracking progress against that plan and those task assignments; and good communication among team members, including periodic meetings and published meeting minutes. Project team managers should be experienced managers who know the organization well, who have credibility and respect as leaders and managers, who understand the health care institution's operations and objectives, and who have experience with information technology—preferably, experience with a similar project.

Vendor representatives and consultants may present persuasive arguments for assuming project management roles themselves, but such practices are best avoided, since a manager from outside the institution may attempt to impose his or her objectives in place of those of the institution. Delegation of management responsibility to an outsider, however, is often a tempting alternative for the institution's managers, who may wish to avoid the complex, difficult, and sometimes unwanted responsibility for success, preferring instead that an outsider be held accountable. If managers are so ambivalent about the objectives that an appropriate internal manager is not available to take on a leadership role, it's unlikely that the project will deliver its full benefits to the institution. Instead of hiring an outsider under these conditions, the project should be reassessed and objectives clarified, subsequently proceeding with an internal manager at the helm.

Competent project planning, task assignment, and task scheduling are vital ingredients for project team success. Plans and work should be defined by assigned team members, possibly with the help of guidelines from vendors or consultants. But those guidelines, although useful, should be tailored to each institution's specific objectives.

The project's success also depends on effective communication among project team members. Regularly scheduled project team meetings should be held to provide a formal method of communicating, as team members report progress and status and raise issues for further assignment. Thorough written documents should be prepared as meeting minutes, subcommittees' progress statements, and when appropriate, as findings and recommendations. These written documents should include details that clarify issues, fix responsibilities, differentiate among alternatives, expose flaws and problems, explain justified revisions, and document decisions.

Effective communication among team members is extremely important in managing physicians' participation on project teams. In general, physicians' career accomplishments have been achieved as a result of their individual capabilities and, to some extent, competition with others. They have high levels of confidence, as they should, and they may have some detailed knowledge of computer principles, but they may have little experience in taking responsibility for a part of the cooperative and organized work of a team, and in negotiating procedural changes for the good of the entire health care institution.

Gaining Wide Acceptance of Clear Objectives

Defining clear objectives

Each project's objectives must be clear—and they must be accepted by team members and others throughout the health care institution. To further such understanding and acceptance, it is valuable to begin the project by summarizing the institution's relevant goals and objectives, as stated in its mission statement or long-range plan. The source and description of the project, and other directions approved by the steering committee, should be examined to determine if the project was derived from a well-defined, long-range objective; a more short-term management objective; or a departmental problem or objective—or perhaps it is simply the consequence of vendor marketing.

Depending on the source of the project's initiation, the planning, analysis, evaluation, and system acquisition effort may require different strategies, different communications among team members, and different work assignments. For example, a project derived from a long-term management objective usually is well understood throughout the hospital, and the potential effect of the project on the interdependent work among departments has already been examined. A project stimulated by a recent vendor marketing effort, however, may be well understood and supported by a single department, but its effect on other departments' work may have received no prior analysis and planning.

Objectives of each project should be first prepared in written form and then discussed and modified in project team discussions. These objectives should address specific areas of management concern, such as budget, cost limitations, and cost management. They should also cover other relevant issues, such as changes to the institution's procedures and potential changes to work relationships among departments.

Dependence on the participants' perceptions of the change

In many health care institutions,[29-35] success of the systems acquisition process has depended in part on employees' ability to accept and adapt to change. Change from current processes are uncomfortable and possibly even frightening, and adapting to change requires investment of great effort by the institution's employees. Teamwork and negotiation are critical, especially when systems change the culture or change work at organizational or political boundaries.

Physicians' and nurses' perceptions of, and reactions to, new computer systems are especially critical, and require the attention of the project manager. The reactions of physicians and nurses will depend to a great extent on how much they know about information technology, and on their negative experiences with information technology in the past. In those systems of the past, for example, the clinicians expected the new systems to eliminate paper, or at least to improve their work, but they were burdened instead by duplication of work. Data had to be entered into the computer, but the manual processes had to be continued in parallel. Moreover, PCs arrived on the scene just in time to add to the confusion: users were misled into painful computer systems failures, believing that PC technology would be easier to implement and more useful than it turned out.[36] Furthermore, to add to the perception problem, in a study of professionals' general perceptions of computer technology, researchers concluded that professional people who have little direct exposure to, or experience with, computers have inaccurate perceptions and negative attitudes toward them.[37]

The attitudes and perceptions, both positive and negative, held by team members and other employees will have a significant impact on the success of a system acquisition project. First, on the positive side, "the greater the perceived need . . . and the lower the level of apprehension . . . the greater the likelihood of success."[38] As traditional beliefs and organizational control issues are threatened, "negotiation of these issues, in an informal and ongoing manner . . . is critical to the success of the project."[39] Furthermore, considering employees' potential stress over fear of job downgrading, breakup of work relationships, future reduction in freedom of action, and relocation of power, "the lower the level of stress engendered . . . the lower the level of resistance and the greater the likelihood of success."[40]

Negative views of the changes that a new system may impose tend to generate resistance. This resistance is sometimes beneficial in the sense that it tends to prevent selection of systems and procedures that might be detrimental to the institution.

The more sensitive the project team is to these negative attitudes and perceptions, and the better adapted their practices are to these issues, the less the conflict and resistance.[41] In particular, thorough assessment of current systems and clear proposals for new procedures can change perception and attitudes. Resulting information, skillfully communicated, informs and convinces employees and physicians that the need for change exists and that such change will benefit the institution, thereby overcoming their fears and persuading them to accept the change.

Assessing Current Systems and Procedures

After the project team informs affected employees of intentions to define and select a new information system, existing systems and procedures are meticulously assessed, and the findings documented and widely communicated.[42] Although the project and the potential new information system may have been fully understood and accepted by the steering committee, some potentially affected employees may not clearly perceive which systems and procedures the new system will affect and what potential value might be derived from the change. The assessment process is designed both to evaluate opportunities for change and to widely communicate findings and intentions among the institution's employees. A great deal of learning takes place during these assessment activities.

Assessing current systems and procedures is very important and very complex in health care; the process examines the strengths of existing systems and identifies opportunities for improvements. Health care is a very information-intensive industry, with information created, exchanged, and collected at every step in the patient care cycle. As a by-product, data are also collected for patient accounting and to provide summary information for managing the institution. Carefully identified improvements in procedures and in the information cycles can reduce costs, accelerate work, eliminate potential errors, and make available more relevant and timely information.

During the assessment, data are collected in a variety of ways. Interviews are conducted with managers and employees who have work responsibilities within the work flow being considered for change. Questionnaires, as in Exhibit 6.1, may be distributed for potential users to complete, and responses solicited and then analyzed. Reports and data input documents should be examined. For work that is expected to be automated for the first time, work flow and information flow should be documented on diagrams, to define how these functions should be automated, as illustrated in Figure 6.1. Performance measures of existing computer systems, such as on-line response time, system availability, and system reliability are documented and matched against industry expectations, as in Exhibit 6.2. This could also be

Exhibit 6.1 Sample Portion of Questionnaire for Distribution to Potential System Users

---

The following is part of a survey being conducted so that our hospital can define a comprehensive list of capabilities of a new clinical system. The responses of all of you will be compiled and reviewed prior to specifying our system requirements to prospective vendors of systems.

Physician identification should be entered by (choose one)

- Last name _____
- Numeric code _____
- Either one, optionally ___X___

Data entry should be via (enter 1 through 5 to indicate priority)

- Keyboard ___1___
- Light pen ___4___
- Mouse ___3___
- Touch screen ___2___
- Voice ___5___

Clinical errors in test request should be able to be corrected by (choose all that apply)

- Clerk _____
- Technician-in-charge ___X___
- Supervisor ___X___

Work list format and content should be (choose one)

- Common to all departments _____
- Unique to departments ___X___
- Unique to supervisor level _____

---

collected by questionnaire. Data input controls should be documented and analyzed. Acknowledged problems are documented and analyzed. Unmet system needs and wish lists are collected. Vendor relationships, reputation, and potential future existence in the market are documented and analyzed. Operating and other recurring costs should be collected and analyzed.

Although the assessment process looms very complex, an excellent starting point is to document data elements and data cycles, as shown in Exhibit 6.3. This again may be accomplished by questionnaire. Data input and output cycles are tangible processes with which most users of current systems are familiar. These processes can serve as the point of departure for

Figure 6.1   Work Flow and Information Flow for
Physical Medicine Order Processing

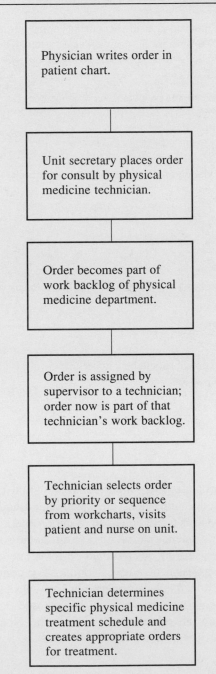

Physician writes order in
patient chart.

Unit secretary places order
for consult by physical
medicine technician.

Order becomes part of
work backlog of physical
medicine department.

Order is assigned by
supervisor to a technician;
order now is part of that
technician's work backlog.

Technician selects order
by priority or sequence
from workcharts, visits
patient and nurse on unit.

Technician determines
specific physical medicine
treatment schedule and
creates appropriate orders
for treatment.

Exhibit 6.2 Sample Comparison of Performance and Capacity Measures
of Existing Systems with Industry Standards and Expectations

Performance Item	Current	Industry Norm or Expectation
Average on-line response time (seconds)	2.7	less than 1.0
No. of scheduled unavailable hours per day	2.0	less than .5
No. of unscheduled stoppages per month	5–10	3 or less
No. of unscheduled unavailable hours per month	5–12	3 or less
Report printing capacity (pages/minute)	10	20
No. of detailed patient records stored	73,000	500,000

performing broader analysis and raising broader issues. For example, documentation of data elements will help identify data elements that should be added, and it will help identify new controls needed on data entry to improve accuracy. It might also identify departmental procedures that are not being properly followed and a need to find mechanisms that will help enforce these procedures. The data and findings should be organized by topic and consolidated in folders that include copies of forms, reports, and diagrams illustrating work and information flow.

Assessing Available Information Technology

Computer technology capability is growing at a startling pace and raising expectations of wondrous automation that will provide great assistance to institutions. But the marketing campaigns of vendors of health care information systems are sometimes guilty of leveraging on these expectations and promoting capability that may not be as useful as potential users are led by them to expect. To offset this strong influence, the project team should gain sound knowledge of any current state-of-the-art computer technology that might be relevant to the system acquisition project. The project team must also assess the difficulty of gracefully migrating from current systems and technology to whatever technology is ultimately selected and acquired.

One method of obtaining information is to attend industry conferences and exhibitions to observe new product demonstrations and make contact with system vendors. Additional information may then be gained through later contacts with these same vendors.

Another method of formally acquiring information is to prepare and distribute a request for information (RFI) to vendors who may later be issued

Exhibit 6.3   Sample Documentation of Existing Data Elements
and Data Cycles

The following is part of a survey being conducted so that our hospital can define a comprehensive list of data elements to be included in our new clinical system. Your responses will be compiled, reviewed by the project team, and then will become part of the specifications given to prospective vendors.

Please review the attached list of data elements. Please enter an **X** in the column "Used" if you currently use that data element in your work. In the column "Future" enter an **N** if you believe the data element is necessary in your work in the new system, **D** if desired, but not necessary, and **I** if you are indifferent.

Data Element	Used	Future
Medical record number	X	N
Patient account number	X	N
Nursing station number	X	N
Room and bed	X	N
Date of birth	X	N
Sex	X	N
Race	—	I
Weight	—	D
DRG code	—	N
Admitting physician name	—	N
Admitting physician number	X	N
Admit date (if inpatient)	X	N
Admit time (if inpatient)	X	N

a request for proposal (RFP). In the RFI, vendors may be asked to provide up-to-the-minute information about their relevant products, including video display screen technology, methods for interconnecting computers, system capacities, languages, data base capabilities, capabilities for uploading and downloading information from and to personal computers, compatibilities with other vendors' products, conformance to industry standards, and their current emphasis on research and development.

After gathering information on vendor products, the project team should conduct site visits to hospitals that are using those products to ensure that information provided in the vendor's response to the RFI is accurate. Site visits to hospitals that are already using information technology successfully can also help project team members to gauge the practicality of new technology.

As a result of these efforts, project team members learn about the life cycles of technologies. Laser printers, for example, are early in their life cycles and beginning to replace impact printers. Impact printers, which are late in their life cycles, are now almost totally displaced by newer technology. Participants learn about the similar life cycles of personal computers, display terminals, display terminal pointing devices, capability for video graphic presentation, and capability to store, transmit, and display clinical diagnostic images.

Armed with hands-on knowledge of available products, the project team is ready to define system requirements and prepare an RFP for distribution to vendors.

Defining Requirements and the Request for Proposal

Transition from assessment to definition

The project team's next step involves using the assessment results to form a clear and precise definition of system requirements—a definition that will evolve into a request for proposal to be sent to vendors. The quality of these definitional activities determines the functional quality of the acquired system and also greatly affects the likelihood of its successful use.[43]

The final document defining system requirements, which will become the RFP, should be written to serve several purposes. It is this document that communicates throughout the institution the final details of system assessment and definition of requirements. This document will also communicate requirements to all vendors equally. Finally, this document should be written so that it, together with the selected vendor's proposal, becomes part of the eventual contract agreement between the institution and the vendor, thereby binding the vendor to what was requested by the customer and promised by the vendor.

Request-for-proposal format

The RFP should provide general information about the institution and the system to be acquired. Overall system objectives should be included, along with a description of the hospital and relevant details of its mission, strategies, and long-term plan. The current computing environment should be described, including an explanation about how the new system must fit in with current processing and delineating any general time phasing among desired functions.

An RFP should also prescribe the format of vendors' responses, so that all proposals contain the same level of information. The RFP should include a specific list of all information that must be provided and all questions that must be answered by the vendor. This ensures that each question is answered directly, not with a general reference to a vendor's reference manual that may supply only an ambiguous answer or require lengthy reading and analysis.

Different types of requirements

The process of defining system requirements is difficult because different departments want to specify and emphasize different requirements. The project team manager must be aware of both the different sources of requirements and the motivations for strong feelings involved. Clinical personnel will want maximum functionality, to ensure greatest usefulness for their clinical work. Personnel in some departments, such as financial analysis or marketing, will want broad capability, not specifically defining the reports and data available, and leaving data access open to ad hoc requests and "what if" analyses of special questions that they must often analyze. Information services representatives will likely seek specific definitions of functions and maximum compatibility with current systems, to reduce both the potential of hidden costs and the burdens of operating and managing interactions and data exchange among incompatible systems. Executive management will be interested in management controls and timely access to a broad data base. Knowledgeable users and people focusing on the institution's best interest will specify justifiable requirements; some others may instead specify unsupportable whims. Credence should be given to the former, while the latter should be required to justify the need for whatever they request.

As requirements are defined, the project manager should also be alert for requirements that are specified by people who are very familiar with computer technology, sometimes called power users. Power users who incorrectly anticipate the value of leading-edge computer technology may firmly but mistakenly specify requirements that few others can understand and, therefore, evaluate. Special efforts must be undertaken to determine whether these leading-edge requirements will, in fact, be useful to, or even useable by, other employees.

One difficulty in defining systems for physicians' use is that the system cannot appear to be limiting their autonomy or their ability to freely change their diagnosis and treatment practices. Such a clinical system must be extremely flexible, thus making it difficult to define specific system requirements.[44]

The degree of detail required to define requirements depends, in large part, on the type of system being defined. If the system is a business transaction system, with broad data input by clerical people in many departments and where up-front precision of the data collection is important, the definition must then precisely specify many details: data elements, data edits, data cycles, ease of use, and specific help screens. If the system is inherently or partially a broad information support system, however, precisely specifying all data elements is not as important.

Defining data elements

A system's data elements and processing characteristics are very interdependent, but data elements offer an easier focal point with which to begin the definition process. Quite simply, they are easier to list and describe than are processing characteristics.

The thorough and correct definition of a system's data elements is extremely important to the success of an acquisition project, and the system's implementation and use within the institution. Research has shown that the likelihood of any information system's success is greatly enhanced by correct decisions on data that should be both included and excluded from the data base.[45] Exclusion is important because a tendency to store great amounts of unimportant data could handicap the system with inappropriate and costly data collection and storage requirements, while perhaps also adding a burdensome increase in data retrieval response times.

This task involves defining and describing the broad list of data elements that must be included in the system, as shown in Exhibit 6.4. The list can be created by analyzing the data elements details collected during the assessment step (Exhibit 6.3), and adding additional data elements to the list. By including this list in the RFP, vendors are required to indicate whether or not each data element is present in their system. Vendors are also able to list additional data elements that are present in their system, allowing easy comparison of proposals. A secondary purpose of preparing the list is to provide an initial focal point for the project team's work, helping team members come to an understanding and agreement first on each data element, and then on the processing that affects or is affected by its presence. The value to the project team of focusing initially on data elements is most important and useful if the system has a broad data scope with many data input sources that are spread out in distance and time. The consolidated list of data elements and descriptions helps project team members understand

and identify with the broad system that each may not be familiar with. As data elements are considered, understood, and accepted by project team members, work emphasis then shifts to related processing capabilities.

Defining necessary processing capabilities

Processing capabilities are the many system functions to enhance the work of people. Processing capabilities include functions to edit data during entry, present data on display screens, perform calculations on data, direct a user at a terminal to perform necessary tasks, print data on reports, and perform analytical tasks such as searching for or sorting certain data.

Exhibit 6.4   Sample Documentation of Required Data Elements

Each vendor is asked to indicate whether the following data elements are contained in their system. Please answer:

A if data element is currently in your system in use in another site,
B if it is available, but not in use,
C if not available, but development is under way for next version,
D if not available, but added at no cost,
E if not available, but can be added at cost to customer, and
F if unavailable and the vendor has no plans to make it available.

You may also add comments as applicable.

Patient-Related Data Elements

Medical record number	A
Patient name	A
Maiden or alias name	D
Date of birth	A
Social security number	A
Sex code	A
Race code	B
Marital status code	A
Employer code	E
Employer name	A
International country code	F

Here, the project team's task is to list all processing functions that the system must include. This task usually can be performed well only if the assessment of existing systems and current technology has been performed well. Furthermore, the task is usually ineffective when project team members fail to invest sufficient effort in defining precisely what the system must do. In this case, they may allow the system to be defined by the vendor product, hoping for a good fit after the system is chosen.

The system's processing capabilities ultimately determine the operations and work flow among the institution's employees, and that work is significantly affected by the quality of the effort invested during system definition. A system definition that includes a thorough, well-defined, and powerful collection of processing capabilities offers a greater likelihood of the project's ultimate success.[46]

Defining modern input and output methods

Processing capabilities that have the greatest impact on operations and work flow are those that affect methods of user access to the system for data input and output. These methods and media for data input and data retrieval—the *computer-human interface* or the *user interface*—also significantly affect the likelihood of an information system's success.

Two different methods of data input and output have evolved, as mentioned earlier in this chapter. The early method of data input, *batch processing,* involves collecting data input in batches and preparing it for a controlled process that defers its entry into the computer system until later, including it in some well-defined cycle, such as daily posting of patient charges. Similarly, batch processing of output involves periodic printing of standard reports, such as daily census reports or monthly departmental financial reports, and scheduled distribution of those reports to users' offices.

The newer method, *on-line processing,* allows transactions to be entered directly into the computer system, usually by an employee in the work area where the transaction actually takes place, such as in order entry processes. Similarly, on-line output allows direct retrieval of data on computer display terminals, such as in direct census inquiry on nursing stations and in registration departments where employees manage patient admissions, transfers, and discharges.

These two methods of processing data are very different and produce far different results. For example, batch processing typically offers greater control over data entry, at the expense of timeliness. In batch processing, data are batched and processed through a person or department that acts as a checkpoint that might impose controls, such as those that prevent fraud in entry of payroll salary increases. However, batch processing results are usually printed on reports that are unavailable until the control processes of the people and computer are complete. If the reports indicate that some data were rejected by the computer or were otherwise incorrect or incomplete, the corrected data must be put through the batch processing cycle once again, again subject to errors and possible corrections.

As a general guideline, if data change infrequently or must be subjected to control audit, some form of batch processing of input data can be used. However, if data change frequently or if infrequent changes must be available instantaneously to all users throughout the hospital, on-line data input processing is better. Additionally, on-line input processing should take place as close to the transaction's actual point of work as possible, similar to the retail industry strategy of automating data entry of transactions at cash registers. Such a strategy may ultimately justify moving data entry of some patient record keeping to the patient's bedside.

For data output, mode of presentation to the ultimate user is vital. More and more information is available in computer systems, and strong dependence may exist between availability of information and an institution's overall performance. Batch processing of output on reports often causes information overload, leading to less use of information even while more is available.[47] On the other hand, information available on-line through user-directed inquiry may go unused because no institutional process directs users to the available data on some frequent cycle.

Regarding output presentation, attention must also be given to data format, the degree of data summarization, availability of detailed information, and the timing of data output cycles. Research has shown, in particular, that the usefulness of computer output to the user in formulating decisions depends significantly on the presentation medium (paper report or video display) and information form (summarized or presented in detail, and availability of graphic presentation).[48]

Research has shown that the effectiveness of a computer system depends more on the human factors involved in end-user methods of input and retrieval of data than on any other computer processing difference. The pivotal role of the data output format requires that managers, instead of delegating this important function, be personally involved.[49] The format of data output must be familiar to users, and it must be tailored to the institution, not requiring strict adherence to what is available in the vendor's system. Output format must additionally be flexible to change and evolution as the system and institution evolve, requiring both powerful report writers, and data inquiry and analysis languages for that purpose. The system must provide end-user computing options, including direct end-user control over a potentially continuing evolution of output formats. Furthermore, the output format requirements definition should specify selected use of laser printing technology, including paper size variations, font variations and sizes, and other options such as underlining and bold printing.

In most hospitals, on-line access should be the preferred method for both input and output, and the system should offer computing options to allow end users to continuously tailor the output to their evolving needs. The resulting system will be more effective because direct access through an on-line mode of operation enhances management use, boosts the system's chances of success, increases users' problem-solving performance, and offers significant improvements in human performance, which often proves to be the single most important factor in successful system use.[50]

Defining capacity requirements

Problems occur when an acquired information system does not have the capacity to process the transaction loads imposed on it. Consequently, attention must be given to defining anticipated processing loads. Statements of capacity requirements ensure that vendor proposals will include computer processing capability sufficient to meet requirements, and that the contract specifically references these details as it defines system acceptance criteria.

Processing loads are often specified in terms of counts of business transactions per time period, such as counts of invoices to be paid or checks to be printed per business cycle, patient registrations per day, or patient orders and tests to be processed per day. Counts that help to predict storage capacities include average daily census, number of physicians on staff, number of employees, number of charges per day, and length of time that patient test results will be stored. From these counts, vendors can extrapolate measures of system capacity and power for their equipment proposals. Also, to aid in determining the number of terminals necessary, system requirements should include a listing or count of the work locations where user interaction is necessary for data input and output.

Defining system availability and failure recovery requirements

Computer systems that are deficient in reliability and availability also reduce the likelihood of the acquired system's success. Here again, success requires careful attention to specifying expectations in these areas. Explicit specifications force vendors to make explicit responses, while also providing details that can later be referenced as acceptance criteria and performance criteria in contracts.

On-line systems should be defined to include availability essentially

24 hours per day. Vendors should be asked to include in their proposals all scheduled functions and other limitations that prevent 24-hour on-line access, and they should be asked to specify the amount of time per day that such processes will prevent on-line access.

Furthermore, the RFP should require that manual downtime procedures be specifically included in the vendor's system procedures and documentation, including any special forms necessary to record transactions manually during periods when the computer system is unavailable.

In addition to these scheduled activities, periodic unscheduled events and system failures also inevitably limit 24-hour access. To cover such occasions, the system requirements should specify that vendor systems' documentation include written instructions for diagnostic steps, recovery, and restart procedures, including controls to prevent mistakes that could make the failure worse. In support of quick system recovery from failure, the RFP requires that vendor proposals describe any redundant resources that are included in the system (such as duplicate copies of certain files or second computer components in standby mode) and detail how they can assist in recovering from different types of system failure. Furthermore, if the computer system is in the patient care loop, collecting data directly from patients or providing data directly for patient care (such as patient monitoring equipment or bedside terminals), the RFP should require that backup computer equipment be immediately available to take over processing in the event of system failure, without inhibiting the work of people in the patient care loop. Computer systems that contain several identical clustered and interconnected items of equipment often provide this capability.

Data security and privacy requirements

Explicit declarations of data security requirements should also be included in the RFP, so that product differences will be immediately evident—and easily evaluated—in vendor proposals. For example, a system's data files must be accessible only under strict controls and only to people with reason to have access. At the same time, those controls must not be so burdensome as to make user access awkward and unuseable by clinical personnel.

Data access guidelines might, for example, allow nursing personnel to gain access to data concerning patients who are on their nursing unit, and under certain conditions to gain access to data on patients being transferred to or from that unit. Physicians should be allowed access to data about their patients and those for whom they have been asked to consult. Some physicians justify gaining access from their homes, but a system that provides that access must not inadvertently expose data to easy access by so-called hackers, computer users attempting to gain unauthorized access. Computer systems provide optional audit trails that report all accesses to certain data items and access under exceptional conditions, such as during certain time periods, so that management may periodically review the reports. Additional information on data access controls and other security is contained in Chapter 8.

Other technical requirements and tools

In addition, other technical requirements and tools are available for many purposes: for prototyping, to improve management and control of software libraries, to improve change management, to reduce system implementation time, and to improve management of the acquired system's operation. Many of these tools are potentially available with the vendor's system, and therefore the requirements should be specified. This ensures that vendor proposals address these requirements, and it provides an easy gauge for comparing the proposals.

Some tools can aid in fitting the system to an institution's evolving needs. For example, prototyping aids allow systems analysts to present simulated display screens to potential users, allowing users to try them and evaluate them before specifications for the real display screen are finalized. Special languages called *application development systems* also provide methods of quickly developing—and changing—display screens. An application development system may also be used as a prototyping aid.

Data base systems and their associated data dictionaries allow the list of data elements and their descriptions to be embedded in the system. Such embedded dictionaries can be referenced directly by tools such as application development systems.

Software utilities can be used to sort data, produce daily backup copies of data, and recover data that is damaged and partially intact. They can also analyze programs to detect flaws in logic before testing and to prepare test data automatically for new modules before they are used.

Library management systems facilitate control of the software program library and also track changes as new versions of system software supersede old versions. Additional tools can compare software modules to detect differences between old and new versions.

In addition, the vendor should be asked to specify the computer language used in all programs. Modern versions of languages provide more capability, both in the current system and in its adaptability for upgrading. Some languages will facilitate future use of important enhancements to video screen displays, improving the computer-human interface. Other languages are more English-like, making it easier for customer or vendor staff to diagnose problems or to enhance systems.

Of course, the source code must be available to be read by both vendor and hospital personnel. The contract should require that the vendor make the source code available so that program errors can be diagnosed, problems can be corrected, and, if necessary, enhancements can be made. This precludes problems if, in the future, the vendor fails to make corrections or refuses to acknowledge problems. The possibility of vendor business failure is an added justification for obtaining access to the source code. If the vendor declares bankruptcy, for example, creditors may seize the vendor's assets— and the source code may be the vendor's only valuable asset. Creditors probably will not be sensitive to the plight of customers, and they may make the source code unavailable. Some vendors escrow their source code to solve this problem, but such a solution is unacceptable. The escrowed version is not only likely to differ from the current version or the version that each customer is using, but legal action by the creditors may also prevent customers from obtaining copies of the source code from an escrow agent.

Defining timing and phasing

Change is frightening, difficult, and costly in terms of its staff-hour requirements. Even with the availability of modern software packages, a fairly large and complex health care institution cannot be converted to new systems in one fell swoop. The system implementation processes must take place in phases.

Even so, the system requirements definition process must define the integrated final system as fully as possible, including the necessary data elements and processing functions. The RFP should also define a specific format and wording by which vendors can declare the timing and phasing of system capabilities to meet the institution's objectives. For system functions that the vendor does not currently have available but that will become available in the future, the RFP should require that the vendor state the timing of the potential future availability. For example, a vendor may be instructed to state the system's future capabilities in terms such as "being developed and scheduled for the next version," "being developed and scheduled for a future version," "planned for a future version but not being developed," and "unavailable and unplanned."

Furthermore, an institution faces great risk by choosing a replacement strategy that totally scraps an existing system and completely replaces it. A safer strategy relies on an evolutionary, phased process that adds and substitutes selected new functions within the framework that currently exists. Evolutionary change must be planned and controlled. Plans should designate points in the future as milestones for changing the system, and management should guide the institution toward each new milestone much as a large ship would be carefully steered.

Because all future needs simply cannot be defined, continuing customization will undoubtedly be necessary. Planned phasing should, therefore, be directed initially toward functions that are most well understood and defined. Users will become more familiar with those system functions, refine their judgments, and consequently make better judgments and decisions about future customization.

Interfaces and integrations among new and existing processes

Research has shown that sound system integration results in increased chances of success.[51] Integrated interconnections among systems provide users with coordinated and blended access to their institution's information systems functions.

There are hidden costs to an institution's poorly integrated, awkward, and risky interfaces among systems. Individual segments of information systems, although suited to the requirements of different eras and difficult to integrate, must be well integrated. If not, poor quality interfaces may invalidate data, or at least discredit it, since manual processes at the point of interface may be inconsistent and unpredictable from cycle to cycle. For example, revenue data passed from the patient accounting process to the monthly financial reporting process may not have compatible data fields for storing cost centers and revenue accounts. Manual processes, necessary for interpretations, might be inconsistent from month to month.

Computerized interfaces that automatically pass data among systems are especially susceptible to failure, because these interfaces are triggered by events such as registrations or completions of patient test results. These interfaces should conform to existing industry standards, such as requiring a consistent number of allowable alphabetic characters in a patient's last name, so that the data can exist in the same form in all systems. Without such standards, time-consuming and costly intellectual work must be undertaken to define specific methods for handling different requirements, such as when a patient name is transferred from one system to another, possibly by truncating a name or adding blank characters to it. Furthermore, the selected new system should allow flexibility to future change, so that an old system or interface can be "unplugged" and a newer one substituted without too much difficulty.

Standards and de facto standards for interfaces are slowly evolving in the health care information industry. Some standards have been established through consensus among interested parties, and some have been established as a result of vendors' leadership in the marketplace. In fact, a single vendor's strong marketing position may dominate a market and, therefore, establish a standard. For example, the early IBM PC and early PC software vendors established many of the standards for the personal computer market. More recently, in the health care information systems marketplace, several vendors and customers have formed work groups to establish specific standards for software interfaces among systems.

The RFP should require vendors to describe all interfaces that are included in, or affected by, their proposal. The vendor proposal should include descriptions both of data elements that must be transferred to the system through an interface and of data elements that are available for automatic transfer to another system. The vendor should also describe methods of transferring data among systems (often called *protocols*), timing and frequency of data transfer, and possible controls that could be imposed on data transfer among systems.

Evaluating and Ranking Vendor Proposals

Comparing vendors' responses with RFP requirements

The purpose of the proposal evaluation process is to compare the requirements defined in the RFP with the details of proposals received from vendors, determining how well each vendor's proposal meets the requirements. During this evaluation, many details must be consolidated and compared. This requires worksheets comparing details collected from all vendor proposals, and it demands well-organized and well-documented effort among many people.

Selection criteria should be specified prior to the evaluation, especially basic requirements that absolutely must be met. In particular, the project team should decide, for each processing or data element requirement, whether that requirement is absolutely necessary in the initial system; required, but could be deferred to a later phase or version of the system; or preferred, but not necessary.

Evaluation checklists are valuable aids in evaluating vendor proposals, site visits, and the vendor corporations. These checklists should be prepared and standardized before vendor proposals are received. A typical checklist, such as that shown in Exhibit 6.5, would list evaluation criteria in the left column, while reviewers' evaluations are entered on the right. Evaluations should be conducted and documented even if project team reviewers believe that one vendor clearly has a better product. This formality convinces all interested parties that the evaluation process was objective and not flawed by personal preferences. The evaluation should encompass services and support proposed by the vendor, including documentation provided, training, installation assistance, warranties, methods and periods of acceptance, and maintenance support.

Exhibit 6.5   Sample Vendor Evaluation Checklist to Evaluate Responses to RFPs

Evaluation Criteria	Max Score Allowed	Systems X	Y	Z
Capabilities (40%)				
1. State-of-the-art technology	40	30	25	15
2. Help screens	10	5	0	5
3. Medical decision support	30	5	5	8
⋮				
System performance/management (20%)				
1. Functioning in another similar site	15	12	9	3
2. Built-in backup recovery	5	5	5	5
3. Flexibility to continued change	20	10	12	10
⋮				
Vendor reputation and support (20%)				
1. Financial status	15	12	8	8
2. Installation team	15	8	8	8
3. Ongoing upgrades	10	7	7	8
⋮				
Cost (20%)				
1. Purchase/license fee	20	12	7	12
2. Ongoing maintenance cost	10	8	9	7
3. Future price protection	10	3	5	3
⋮				
TOTALS	200	117	100	92

As the tabulations for vendor proposals are completed and consolidated, each vendor's unmet requirements should be individually analyzed, as should each major difference among the differing vendor proposals. This analysis will determine if an unmet requirement is so vital that the vendor's proposal is consequently unacceptable. When such a condition is discovered, and details are verified with a vendor representative, that vendor proposal should be removed from further consideration. Other unmet requirements and major differences should simply be tabulated and consolidated for future reference while ranking the vendor proposals.

System integration, the hospital culture, and human factors

The achievement of manageable integrated systems is a critical objective for the project team. Consequently, in deciding among the competing vendor proposals, evaluators on the project team must determine how suitable the vendor's proposed system will be for interconnection and integration with existing systems and procedures.

Evaluators must judge how well the new system can be tailored to the hospital's existing culture, management style, and terminology. The evaluators must also determine how much change the hospital would be required to undertake to accommodate system functions that cannot be tailored to the hospital's requirements.

The evaluators must also assess the quality of the computer-human interface, including the clarity and usefulness of the video display screens, the extent of conformance to emerging standards for presentation on video display screens, and the breadth and ease of use of available data retrieval and data analysis options.

The evaluators must also take the perspective of computer production services management, determining how well integrated operations of old and new systems will be. Furthermore, expecting an operational mix possibly including several different vendors' products, the evaluators must determine how manageable the processes of diagnosing and correcting errors will be. In addition, the evaluators must determine whether points of interconnection among systems are specific and obvious enough that problems can be identified with the vendor whose product failed—or to what extent the hospital will be exposed to the ambiguity and frustration of problems occurring beyond vendors' normal solution procedures. If the points of interconnection do not allow easy identification of vendor problems, the several vendors' maintenance representatives may blame each other and avoid problems that do occur. At best, they must undertake complex coordination with each other, requiring far more time to solve the problem than would ordinarily be necessary.

Finally, taking the perspective of the project team that will be assigned to implement the system, the evaluators must determine how extensive and difficult it will be to convert existing computer data files to those required in the new system.

System age and life cycle: Flexibility and the future

In this era of increasingly rapid technological change, even the best planned and managed computer software products often lag behind the state of the art in at least some of their system capabilities. In fact, a vendor system usually includes many capabilities: some capabilities may be very new and use modern technology, some may be more mature and use older technology, and some may be obsolete. Modern capabilities that provide added and useful functions could also risk using technology that is not fully tested. Older, more mature capabilities offer sound and tested functionality but may lack the power and usefulness that more modern technology offers. Dependence on software that has been in use for many years exposes customers to the threat of maintenance support that may be withdrawn or very difficult to administer.

Similarly, computer hardware capabilities are changing quickly. New generations of equipment are always faster, smaller, cheaper, and more reliable, and they have greater capacity for storage, consume less electrical power, and provide enhanced user capabilities. Older generations, on the other hand, are more fully tested and predictable.

The project team must evaluate vendor products and determine the life cycle position for each of the major software and hardware capabilities and technical characteristics. Six typical life cycle positions exist:

1. Newly conceived and relatively untested

2. New technology, not proven, in early use by one or very few institutions that are leading with this technology

3. Successfully used by institutions leading within this technology, now in use by some follower institutions

4. Modern technology in wide industry use

5. Mature technology in wide use, but more modern technology is being conceived and tested in some institutions

6. Mature technology, but newer technology has successfully displaced it in many institutions

The evaluators on the project team should determine which of these six life cycle descriptions apply to each major functional capability listed in the RFP (for example, processing options for outpatients or comprehensiveness of stored medical record data) and each technical characteristic (for example, use of local area networks or capability for uploading and downloading data from and to personal computers).

For both software and hardware, however, it is quite difficult for vendors to plan and continually upgrade their systems through the steps of a systems life cycle. Some vendors acknowledge the need to conscientiously plan and manage this upgrading, making future product extensions and replacement versions that are compatible with older versions of their products. In these cases, product extensions are issued with version numbers that identify which version is the most modern version and which version the customer is currently using. A vendor following a strategy of providing continuous and compatible upgrades allows customers the advantage of preserving their investment in acquired hardware and software. By planning and managing gradual and continuous product upgrading, customers can continue to make use of state-of-the-art technology over a period of time.

Unfortunately, other vendors fail to acknowledge the need for continuity. These vendors issue new and replacement technology every few years, essentially destroying their customers' investment in the original technology. This forces customers to reinvest the cost and effort necessary to replace both hardware and software—only to catch up with state of the art for yet another short-lived period.

To ensure future continuity, the project team must determine, for each proposal, which type of product upgrading strategy the vendor proposes and, judging from the vendor's experience, which type of strategy is likely in the future.

Underlying technology and capacity

The underlying computer technology platform is extremely important, requiring detailed analysis during the selection of a system. This underlying technology could be a single large mainframe computer, one or more minicomputers, or a network of several different types of computers. In fact, stated requirements may be met with no more than microcomputers that are networked together. Consequently, the project team must analyze vendor proposals to determine the differences in underlying technology, and how well each alternative meets system requirements. The assistance of an outside consultant may be required if several different architectures are proposed, especially if some alternatives rely on leading-edge networking technology.

Pinpointing hardware's proper capacities is also a vital factor in system selection. *Proper capacity* adequately meets requirements but does not provide more capacity than needed. Chosen systems must additionally be capable of orderly growth in capacity to accommodate potential increased work loads in the future.

Undersized equipment causes unacceptably long on-line response times and processing that lags behind schedule. These two consequences will likely cause the project's failure.

By the same token, it is equally inappropriate to purchase computer equipment that has more capacity than required, because the extra capacity will go unused and wasted. Some vendors encourage customers to purchase extra capacity, expecting the extra capacity to allow the vendor to market added software capability later. The risk to this approach is that, since the added capacity is available, the vendor's marketing influence could lead to acquisition of systems outside the steering committee's priorities and executive management control. Also, as the vendor subtly markets software enhancements to make use of the unused capacity, customers might also be tempted to bypass the benefits of a formal competitive system acquisition process.

Instead, a good selection is a system architecture that allows initial selection of specific models of computer equipment, and gradual upgrading in steps, at modest prices, as increased capacity is required in the future. Another good alternative is a technology that allows for the purchase of additional computers that can be interconnected to meet the growing capacity requirements by sharing the work load.

The vendor: Market position, financial stability, and people

Each vendor corporation must also be carefully evaluated, because vendors' reputations and commitments to customer support vary widely. Small vendors may provide special support attention in certain situations, such as for a new customer or with a critical new product, but they may provide only marginal support at other times. Large vendors have greater resources available and, possibly, more industry experience. Because of their large size, however, these vendors may have difficulty managing processes that deliver that support when and where it is needed.

Each vendor's market position should be carefully examined to determine current stability, and future likelihood of continued existence and ability to provide product upgrades. Both large and small vendors potentially could provide future product upgrades that are at the leading edge of technology. For example, large vendors, which usually invest more in research and development, potentially are more able to deliver high-quality upgrades in the future. On the other hand, the efforts of small vendors may be more focused, resulting in higher-quality creative work and quicker and better future product upgrades. Each vendor's financial stability should also be evaluated, a task best accomplished by obtaining and carefully examining their published financial statements.

Additionally, some attempt should be made to assess the vendor by evaluating its representatives: the vendor's employees with whom the project team works. Are they ethical and trustworthy, so that sound working relationships can be developed between the vendor's employees and the institution's employees? Are they competent, or do they rely primarily on lavish marketing entertainment? Are they organized and prepared for meetings, or are their meetings simply general discussions? Are they good business people who will help their companies succeed? Project team members frequently can sense enough from working relationships during the acquisition project to make an accurate vendor evaluation.

Costs

Finally, costs must be reviewed and tabulated. All costs should be analyzed, including equipment, software license, training, installation assistance, travel expenses for vendor employees, and hardware and software maintenance support. As costs are tabulated, it is also important to pinpoint the length of the initial warranty period and, as a result, how soon after system installation future maintenance payments are due.

Special attention should be given to conditions under which unexpected extra costs could be incurred. For example, if the vendor's training department is a revenue center, as opposed to a support center, there is some likelihood that the vendor's training department will have some incentive for bringing about conditions that may increase the costs of training. To avoid such a situation, the contract should impose very rigid controls on expenses beyond those contracted for or otherwise expected.

As costs are analyzed, the project team should also be alert for other unexpected costs that are related to facility preparation: renovation, installation of special electrical power and air-conditioning, cabling for computer terminals, consulting and legal costs of a difficult contract negotiation process, insurance, computer paper and special forms (especially costly multipart forms), and other supplies.

Site visits and user reference

Site visits provide an opportunity for project team members to visit locations where the vendors' systems are already installed. These visits to customer locations, plus other reference checks with current users, usually generate useful information about the vendors' products and customer support.

Site visits are usually arranged by the vendor, whose purpose is to show their product in the best possible light. However, the project team should impose some conditions to ensure that the visit provides as much objective, useful information as possible. The visit should be made by project team representatives from diverse departments of the hospital. An agenda for the visit should be planned and controlled so that project team members are able to question system users in many departments of the visited institution. Otherwise, the site visit may become little more than another vendor marketing presentation, with a simple tour of only those departments that provide favorable impressions.

One project team objective during site visits is to determine if products perform as specified in the vendor proposal. Another objective is to question host customer personnel about details and problems of installation, conversion, training, system performance and capacity, and continuing maintenance support. Project team members will learn much by comparing these details with those in the vendor's proposal.

Keep in mind that vendors choose customer sites that are likely to provide the best impression and where the project team will hear the most positive comments possible. In addition, some customers are simply reluctant to make negative comments about a system during a site visit. Some vendors, for example, pay customers for conducting site visits; other customers may have a royalty interest in the product. It may be wise to ask the host customer if it derives economic benefit from the site visit or from sales of the vendor's products. Current users of a vendor's system could also have additional reasons for withholding negative comments about the system. They may feel that such comments reflect unfavorably on their decision to acquire the system or on their ability to manage its operation and use.

Other user reference checks are very useful to balance the subjectivity of site visit customers who are chosen by the vendor and are likely to provide only positive comments about the vendor's products. Even before conducting site visits, project team members should contact other customers of the vendor, possibly through professional societies or health care industry relationships. These customers often provide objective information on the product's performance and on the quality of vendor relationships and support. Relevant questions may be posed in a telephone interview or on a site visit conducted without vendor participation.

User groups are also a good source of information about a vendor's products. In fact, the very existence of an active user group is a positive indicator about the vendor, its products, and its customers. First, the existence of the user group indicates that the vendor's products are used widely and that the vendor and its customers invest effort in the user group's organization and continued functioning. The user group also provides a forum through which customers can not only obtain assistance and other useful contact, but also influence the vendor to upgrade its products.

If possible, project team representatives may want to attend a user group meeting during the evaluation and selection period. Such a meeting provides ample opportunity to contact existing customers. Additionally, the user group meeting agenda provides valuable information about past and future evolution of the vendor's products.

Opening Contract Negotiations

After vendor proposal evaluations have been completed and the finalists have been ranked, discussions on business arrangements and potential contract agreements should begin with the vendor that is ranked highest. Copies of standard industry contracts, possibly from other vendors, should be reviewed. However, the initial discussions among project team and vendor representatives should focus on details of the business arrangement in which the institution is interested. In this area, understanding and agreement by all parties is vital.

As a general warning before starting the discussions of this section, the advice of competent legal counsel is crucial in this contracting process. The concepts involved are very complex, and the contract could have significant economic and legal implications for the hospital.

Agreeing on the general business arrangement

Contract negotiations can be extremely difficult, especially if the parties involved see results in terms of winning and losing. In fact, the objective of the contract negotiating process must be to strike a clear agreement on the business arrangement and on the responsibilities of all parties involved.

While the final contract must state the business agreement in legal terms, an excellent starting point is to define the general terms of the business deal in a working document that is not necessarily signed by anyone. Later, the contract can be drafted based on details of this working document. The working document should briefly describe all important points, such as major technical details, the proposed time period for system installation, services the vendor will provide, services the customer will provide, approximate costs, interconnection and integration objectives, and the general sharing of risk of failure among the parties. The document should also include future considerations, such as subsequent software versions that will contain functions not included in the vendor's current version of the system.

The importance of clear terminology

Information technology contracts require substantial reference to special technical terms, not all of which are well understood. Therefore, the first requirement of an information systems contract is to define all technical terms clearly and thoroughly.

The contract should contain clear definitions for all terms that are critical to determining conformance to the contract, such as "completion of installation," "first use," "beginning of parallel operation," and "system acceptance." Contract conformance should be associated with measurable events that are obvious to both parties. Conformance based on concepts that are known and controlled only by the vendor are not acceptable, such as "completion of software loading." In such a case, no one but the vendor may really know if this is, in fact, complete. Conformance should be based instead on milestones such as "first use in first designated nursing station."

The concept of a software license

Software acquisition is usually governed by a software license. This license grants perpetual use of the software to customers for a fee, but it does not transfer ownership of the software. It is important that the license specify perpetual use; otherwise, future use could be subject to new and surprising conditions. Many vendors may also charge an optional annual maintenance fee for providing assistance in diagnosing and correcting errors and for providing future upgrades at no additional charge. Payment of such an annual charge, however, should not be a condition for continued use of the software.

To prevent difficulties concerning software ownership, the contract should include the vendor's declaration that it has the right to market the software. Without this protection, a third party—perhaps another vendor, or even another hospital—may claim ownership of the software and take legal steps to prevent others from using it. Contract provisions must ensure the customer's continued right to use the software even in such an event.

Another major ownership and usage question involves intellectual rights to any future enhancements that a customer makes using its own resources or that a customer conceives, designs, or pays the vendor to develop solely for the customer. Some vendors attempt to insist that all future enhancements, made by anyone, automatically become the vendor's property. While vendors have some logic to support this strategy, the customer must carefully consider whether such a statement should be part of a contract that, once signed, will affect all future enhancements. For example, a reasonable and fair business agreement might provide that work performed by the customer's own staff is its intellectual property, and that the vendor cannot take this property and sell it or give it to another customer. The initial agreement might also state that ownership of enhancements that are performed with the vendor's assistance at the customer's expense may become the property of either or both, depending on contract details that are agreed to at the time the enhancements are identified and commissioned.

The vendor's edge in contract negotiations

Contract negotiations are in some ways inherently stacked in the vendor's favor. Vendor representatives, for example, negotiate contracts frequently, while customers face such contractual issues much less often. Also, a vendor may start the negotiating process by simply offering its standard contract for signature, initially balking at any significant modification or extension. This balking may come either as part of the vendor's strategy, or simply because the vendor's bureaucracy is so entrenched that exceptions to the standard contract are seldom approved. Furthermore, while balking, the vendor can usually determine which project team members most want the use of the package, possibly physicians or other caregivers. When the vendor signals subtly to that party that the customer's negotiators are holding up the process, even more pressure is put on these negotiators to agree to the vendor's terms.

Failure to bargain seriously for a clear and fair business deal, however, is a missed opportunity. The customer should assume that the vendor's standard, preprinted contract serves the vendor well, otherwise the vendor wouldn't use it. The customer should appeal for and work toward a fair and clear business agreement.

Contract assurances and the concept of the vendor at risk

The vendor's standard contract usually states conditions under which equipment is to be purchased and software is to be licensed, but it frequently does not state what is to happen if major flaws or failures occur. With the fast-paced innovation that characterizes information systems today, great risk of failure does exist, especially if the product is relatively new and few people have experience with the technology. The contract must be amended to state options and responsibilities should these failures or performance problems arise.

Contract wording that acknowledges potential failures and resulting responsibilities is usually avoided by the vendor because it raises unpleasant issues: namely, vendor assurances, customer or vendor responsibilities, and the assumption of the risk of failure. The contract should definitely state what options are available to the customer if the technology does not work properly, how long the customer is expected to endure while the vendor attempts a remedy, how long the vendor must endure a poorly managed customer implementation process, and how the risk of failure will be shared by customer and vendor.

Purchase and lease alternatives, pricing, and payments

The contract must also define methods of financing the acquisition and the timing of payments. The decision between purchasing or leasing equipment may have major financial effects. Pricing and protection against future price increases, and the timing of payments, also have major budget consequences and must be understood and clearly defined.

The accounting consequences of a lease should be thoroughly analyzed by competent financial accounting personnel. A lease carries an implicit cost of capital, which can be estimated fairly easily from the amounts and timing of the proposed lease payments by calculating what interest rate the institution would be paying for the privilege of leasing. If this interest rate is higher than the prime rate or other financing rates, other financing options should probably be pursued. The length of time that the institution expects to use the equipment and the equipment's expected useful life should also be considered. If the institution expects to use the equipment for only a short time, or if there is risk that the equipment may become obsolete because near-term new products will be better and cheaper, leasing may be an attractive alternative that limits risk of investment loss in the purchase. Furthermore, Medicare reimbursement in the form of credit for capital pass-through might also affect the accounting decision to lease or purchase.

The timing of payments should be carefully considered. The vendor should not expect payment at the time of contract signing; payments should instead be made dependent on value received. For example, the contract should specify major measurable events of system implementation, and payments to the vendor should be made based on successful completion of those events.

Some contract attention should be given to situations where one vendor, possibly a software or leasing company, is to be paid charges for support services that will be provided by another party, such as a hardware maintenance vendor. For example, charges may be contractually due to one vendor for services expected from another vendor; but if, for some reason, the intermediate vendor does not, in turn, make payments to the other vendor, services on which the customer depends may be withheld.

Contracting for future services and options

After signing the contract and successfully installing a system, the vendor may no longer be quite as accommodating to the customer. The contract should, therefore, include some details establishing minimum future performance levels. For example, the maintenance contract should probably include both a statement guaranteeing timely vendor response to problems and some penalty for not meeting that minimum threshold.

The contract must also address other options and conditions that will occur in the future. It might state that the vendor must provide for automatic and timely system upgrades that could be required by future changes in health care regulations, such as for Medicare reimbursement. The contract should also state what options are guaranteed or otherwise available at points of transition in the business transactions. For example, the maintenance and support contract usually is renewable in annual increments. It may be prudent to include provisions in the contract to protect against unreasonable price increases by a vendor that knows customers have little option but to renew.

Other contract details

The contract will contain many other details that must be defined and possibly negotiated. Several people, including legal counsel, should read through the contract carefully and note all details that are not clearly described, understood, and accepted. For instance, some standard contract language allows the vendor to terminate a contract automatically under certain conditions, such as if a customer allows confidential vendor material to be released and obtained by a competitor. However, this language would be equally useful to the vendor, and less threatening to the customer, if it were changed to prevent the vendor from invoking such termination without prior notice and opportunity for the customer to provide a remedy. In any event, once the customer acquires a system, the customer's success might depend on continued and uninterrupted system use. Therefore, the customer might be wise to scrutinize the wording of all contract clauses that would allow the vendor to terminate the contract.

System acceptance should also be addressed in the contract. Successful acceptance requires that several cycles of events successfully take place. Consequently, acceptance is not a single event occurring at a single point in time. Instead, it involves a period of time and must usually continue through at least one monthly cycle.

Much contract wording deals with legal details that legal counsel must evaluate and approve, including liability, method of resolution and jurisdiction for legal action, patent and copyright details, confidentiality of vendor intellectual property, and confidentiality of customer data and patient records. For example, with regard to clinical systems with computer-assisted diagnostic or treatment capabilities, defective or malfunctioning computer systems raise questions of liability.[52] The extent of the vendor's risk should be negotiated and specified in the contract.

Contracts should cover logistics of use. Contracts should state the conditions under which the source code will be made available to the customer, and they should provide for optional use of the system in another facility if an emergency requires computer operation at an alternate site. If the institution is a multientity institution, the contract also should state any conditions for use by the several entities.

Contracts might additionally prevent recruiting of employees of and by either party. Such a cause can prevent potential conflict of interest for employees who might shift their loyalty to the other institution while still entrusted with responsibilities by their original employer.

Balancing Caution and Optimism

Management must closely monitor the activities of project teams assigned to system acquisition projects to balance optimism and caution throughout the entire system acquisition process. The project teams define requirements under the optimistic assumption that they will be met by one or more vendor proposals. After making that assumption, however, the project teams must carefully and cautiously evaluate vendor proposals to avoid being naively led to acquire a system and attempt a project that is infeasible, uneconomical, or too difficult for the institution's users. A system acquisition project is a trying experience for both vendor and customer personnel—whether the effort succeeds or fails. A proper balance of caution and optimism provides the best opportunity for success.

Notes

1. V. C. Pivnicny and J. G. Carmody, "Criteria Help Hospitals Evaluate Vendor Proposals," *Healthcare Financial Management* 43, no. 6 (June 1989): 38, 40, 42.
2. P. Ein-Dor and E. Segev, *A Paradigm for Management Information Systems* (New York: Praeger Publishers, 1981), pp. 103–30.
3. Ibid.
4. Ibid.
5. Ibid.
6. Pivnicny and Carmody, "Criteria Help Hospitals."

7. M. J. Manfredi, "Careful Planning of Software License Agreements Deters Disputes," *Healthcare Financial Management* 43, no. 4 (April 1989): 36, 38, 40.
8. A. Lupovitch, "The Hospital Information System: A Physician's Perspective," *Health Progress* 67, no. 8 (October 1986): 29–31, 62.
9. S. E. Jacobs, "Facilities Management of Hospital Data Processing," in *Information Systems for Patient Care,* ed. B. I. Blum (New York: Springer-Verlag, 1984), pp. 187–95.
10. Manfredi, "Careful Planning."
11. G. J. Mann, "Managers, Groups, and People: Some Considerations in Information Systems Change," *Healthcare Management Review* 13, no. 4 (1988): 43–48.
12. Pivnicny and Carmody, "Criteria Help Hospitals."
13. Lupovitch, "The Hospital Information System."
14. B. F. Minard, "Growth and Change Through Information Management," *Hospital & Health Services Administration* 32, no. 3 (August 1987): 307–18.
15. F. J. Turisco and A. P. Mackin, "Leahy Clinic: Implementing an Order Entry and Result Reporting System for Cardiac Testing," *Computers in Healthcare* (April 1989): 27, 30–32, 34.
16. A. G. Watlington, "Benefits Realization at Mercy Memorial Results in a Changed Organizational Culture," *Computers in Healthcare* (August 1989): 26–29, 32.
17. D. H. McConnell and M. A. Brenner, "HIS: The Clinician's Role," *Computers in Healthcare* (June 1989): 20–22, 24.
18. Ein-Dor and Segev, *A Paradigm,* pp. 103–30.
19. Mann, "Managers, Groups, and People."
20. Minard, "Growth and Change."
21. Watlington, "Benefits Realization."
22. McConnell and Brenner, "HIS."
23. S. Denger et al., "Implementing a Clinical Information System," *Journal of Nursing* 18, no. 12 (1988): 28–34.
24. N. M. Lorenzi and E. B. Marks, "University of Cincinnati Medical Center: Integrating Information," *Bulletin of the Medical Library Association* 76, no. 3 (July 1988): 231–36.
25. Denger et al., "Implementing a Clinical Information System."
26. T. Taylor, "Rx for Computer Angst," *Healthweek* (October 23, 1989): 21–27.
27. C. Safran et al., "Role of Computing in Patient Care in Two Hospitals," *M.D. Computing* 8, no. 3 (May/June 1989): 141–48.
28. W. F. Bria, "Physician Involvement in PCIS Creates Enthusiasm," *U.S. Healthcare* (November 1989): 34.
29. Minard, "Growth and Change."
30. Mann, "Managers, Groups, and People."
31. C. Dunbar, "It's Not Me, It's We," *Computers in Healthcare* (Spring 1989): 17–20.
32. L. W. DiGiulio and T. K. Zinn, "Actualizing System Benefits—Part III," *Computers in Healthcare* (July 1988): 26–28.

33. Denger et al., "Implementing a Clinical Information System."
34. McConnell and Brenner, "HIS."
35. Lorenzi and Marks, "University of Cincinnati Medical Center."
36. B. Neuman and R. G. Bonstein, Jr., "Strategic Information Systems: Opportunities of the 1990's," *Dimensions in Health Care* no. 89–3 (December 1989): 2.
37. E. Zoltan-Ford and A. Chapanis, "What Do Professional Persons Think about Computers," in *Use and Impact of Computers in Clinical Medicine,* ed. J. G. Anderson and S. J. Jay (New York: Springer-Verlag, 1987), p. 65.
38. Ein-Dor and Segev, *A Paradigm,* p. 189.
39. Lorenzi and Marks, "University of Cincinnati Medical Center."
40. Ein-Dor and Segev, *A Paradigm,* pp. 196, 203.
41. Ibid., pp. 203, 205.
42. G. Kolenaty, "Hospital Information Systems Planning," in *Information Systems for Patient Care,* ed. B. I. Blum (New York: Springer-Verlag, 1984), pp. 147–64.
43. Ein-Dor and Segev, *A Paradigm,* pp. 103–30.
44. H. D. Banta, "Embracing or Rejecting Innovation: Clinical Diffusion of Health Care Technology," in *Use and Impact of Computers in Clinical Medicine,* ed. J. G. Anderson and S. J. Jay (New York: Springer-Verlag, 1987), p. 149.
45. Ein-Dor and Segev, *A Paradigm,* pp. 104, 118.
46. Ibid., p. 106.
47. Ibid.
48. Ibid., pp. 106–12, 119.
49. Ibid.
50. Ibid., pp. 123, 125–26.
51. Ibid., pp. 127–29.
52. A. W. Hafner et al., "Computers in Medicine: Liability Issues for Physicians," *International Journal of Clinical Monitoring and Computing* 6 (1989): 185–94.

7

SYSTEMS: IMPLEMENTATION AND INSTITUTIONAL CHANGE

Although the system selection process is fraught with alternatives and critical choices, an even greater number of vital technical and customization decisions will be made during the system implementation process. Success depends on the results of implementation decisions and activities just as much as on the thorough definition of requirements and careful selection of a good information system. Realizing the full benefits of a successful implementation project requires executive commitment and leadership, careful planning of institutional change, competent and cooperative work by project teams, sound technical decisions, sound customization judgments, and capable management.

Managing the Implementation Team

Guiding Inevitable Change

Any system implementation project demands good management of complex and dreaded change. In fact, new information systems often are important catalysts for institutional change, and the system to be implemented may serve as the main component of a new institutional objective. In addition, some hospitals have determined that system implementation may also be used to focus scrutiny on, and improve, other procedures that are peripherally linked to those that automation will directly affect.[1-5] The management challenge, therefore, is to take full advantage of the implementation project as a tool for improving quality and efficiency of procedures as broadly as possible throughout the health care institution.

Executive and Management Support

The commitment of executive and management support is essential in all phases of planning, acquiring, and implementing information systems, but management participation during the implementation process is especially crucial. Management support plays a vital role both in guiding the health care institution through change and in reaping the benefits planned in earlier phases. Some researchers hypothesize that lack of commitment and involvement from management is a major cause of failure for information systems projects.[6]

Successful system implementations occur when executive and management commitment is strong and actively communicated throughout the hospital. The best starting point is for executives to formally tell management, employees, and physicians that the hospital is committed to the information system; they can then begin delegating specific responsibilities that will lead to success. Their participation—and dedication—will motivate others to support the system and the procedural changes involved.

Communicating Objectives and Benefits

Personnel who are well informed about a change to a new system, its objectives, and its benefits are less apprehensive and less resistant to the change. Consequently, any project's chances of success are enhanced by effective communication. Employees and physicians are more likely to perceive the need for change when they have a detailed understanding of the effort it will require and the benefits it will bring. Experience has shown that success in translating management goals into working systems is tied directly to the degree and effectiveness of specific goal definition.[7] It's also been demonstrated that formal, structured lines of communication between users and implementers tend to reduce conflict and promote success.[8] Finally, early communication is crucial; as in most communication efforts, the first few sentences on the subject may determine the endeavor's outcome.

Even after communicating objectives, establishing perception of need, and achieving acceptance of a new system, management's continued efforts to cultivate hospitalwide understanding facilitate system utilization. Turnover of personnel, for example, necessitates ongoing communication. In addition, change usually breeds more change, creating momentum that may be confusing and threatening to those it affects. Only continued communication maintains an institutional environment in which change can flourish.

The All-Important Project Team

One very important management challenge of system implementation is to manage successfully the efforts of employees, management personnel, and, potentially, physicians working together on the assigned project team.[9] This team ideally includes a diverse mix of representatives from among all personnel that will be affected by the new system.[10] Of the team members, as many as possible should be influential high-level managers, including nurse managers, and in the case of clinical systems, influential physicians. Studies have shown that this strategy both increases their later use of the system and boosts its chances of success.[11,12]

Barriers to effective management of project teams do exist, and successful system implementation requires that they be understood and overcome. For example, many clinical personnel may be new users of information systems, and special learning activities may be necessary to help these people learn so that they may effectively contribute. Moreover, the culture in many hospitals includes partitioned organizational power bases, such as major departments, physician groups, and academic researchers. The resulting fragmentation may strengthen special interests, but it undermines the hospital's ability to accommodate change. The project team manager's vital twofold challenge is to encourage innovative thinking among the diverse participants while at the same time leading them to agreement. Project team members will disagree on many issues, but consensus can only be reached by considering alternative proposals—not by overwhelming the team with the work of a powerful few.

In any system implementation project, it's important to clearly define duties and responsibilities of both implementers and users. The potentially huge investment of time by all potential project participants and ultimate system users pushes the real cost of implementation far higher than the payments to vendors, and careful management of that time and effort controls expenses and keeps productivity high. When the many project team members as well as the many potential users throughout the institution clearly understand their responsibilities, the singularity of purpose that results brings greater acceptance, reduced conflict, and an increased likelihood of success.[13]

Depending on the degree of complexity involved, implementation of a new information system can have several phases that span many months. In these cases, the project team shifts its focus several times—and participants face the stress of lengthy projects from definition of requirements to system installation. Under such conditions, the project manager is often able to maintain participants' enthusiasm by restructuring the team in order to manage differently for different phases of the project's life cycle, each with its own unique work and special activities.

When the process works well, the collective effort of project team members, together with fellow hospital employees who are experts in the institution's work, continuously determine goals that must and can be achieved. When the project team is managed well, it is able to achieve these goals.

Plans, Assignments, and Documentation

As was the case with the project team assigned to select and acquire the system, the system implementation project team functions more effectively when it has a detailed work plan and well-defined task assignments, a good method of tracking progress against the work plan, and a sound method of communicating among team members working on related efforts. A detailed, computerized work plan of tasks and responsibilities, including scheduled milestones and updated as progress is noted or changes are prescribed, provides an excellent method of meeting these requirements. The project team additionally benefits from holding regular scheduled meetings. A comprehensive work plan, such as that shown in Exhibit 7.1, can serve as a portion of the agenda for those meetings, while documented meeting minutes provide communication both to project team members and to others not attending the meetings. Meeting minutes also leave a formal audit trail of the project team's work.

Task management during implementation may pose an even more difficult management challenge than it did in the system acquisition process. The scope of project activities is much wider, with many more people involved, greater dependencies among tasks, and more tasks under way simultaneously. A larger number of choices among alternatives are required during implementation, and the project's success is more exposed to many parties' unchecked decisions and influences. Skillful management of multiple and interdependent activities is crucial. Furthermore, management efforts are focused not only on current and high-priority activities, but also on the future activities to which they lead. Projects leading directly into one another create continuity and synergy.

The Special Needs of Clinical Personnel

New clinical systems—often innovative, complex, and potentially affecting a great number of patient care professionals—will require special attention to the reactions of the clinical personnel affected. Moreover, such systems

Exhibit 7.1   Sample Project Plan that Serves also as a Portion of the Agenda for Meetings of the Project Team

Project: Implementation of Interface between Clinical Lab System and Main HIS Computer System

		Schedule by Week											
		Oct.				*Nov.*				*Dec.*			
Tasks	*Responsible Person(s)*	*1*	*2*	*3*	*4*	*1*	*2*	*3*	*4*	*1*	*2*	*3*	*4*
1.01 Define internal communications definitions for HIS	JAD	X	X										
1.02 Define internal communications definitions for clinical lab system ⋮	JBB	X	X										
2.01 Install hardware necessary on HIS	MDY		X	X	X								
2.02 Install hardware necessary on clinical lab system ⋮	BBS		X	X	X								
3.01 Install interface software on HIS	PMK			X	X	X							
3.02 Install interface software on clinical lab system ⋮	PPJ			X	X	X							
4.01 Test software interconnection in single session	LMT						X	X					
4.02 Test software interconnection in complex session ⋮	HTS								X				
5.01 Define manual controls	LMT						X	X	X	X			
5.02 Verify manual controls ⋮	HML									X			

will probably require a long, phase-by-phase implementation period, further straining the clinicians' understanding and acceptance.

Physicians and nurses are often skeptical of new computer systems, either because of past experiences or poor understanding of information technology, and are likely to be reluctant to invest the extra short-term effort to become familiar with the technology and attempt to use new computerized methods.[14] Hospitals have been successful at overcoming these attitudes by using a special implementation group of physicians and nurses.[15] Clinicians usually are influenced strongly by other clinicians, and these special implementation groups help overcome skepticism and encourage clinicians' use of the system. Clinicians will use the system when they believe that it will be useful.[16]

Educating the Project Team

To ensure smooth implementation, the project team manager must place high priority on enhancing project team members' knowledge of technical and organizational topics on which the implementation may depend. Improved knowledge of these topics leads to better team participation and promotes favorable attitudes, user involvement, and chances of the project's success.[17] Moreover, relevant education ensures that important decisions are not made by persons incapable of understanding the implications of their selections.

Improving Computer Literacy

Some project team members may possess only weak knowledge of complex and changing information technology; furthermore, they may fail to acknowledge that weakness. It is up to the project manager to bring the possibility of inadequate knowledge before the project team, spurring team members' self-assessment and growth in understanding. With sufficient encouragement, participants will recognize that information technology encompasses much more than just the basic computer. It includes telecommunications equipment, local area networks, and automated capabilities to diagnose technical problems and measure system performance.

Project team members can gain computer technology knowledge by attending seminars designed to teach important technical principles to lay persons. Seminars may be arranged on site and tailored to the audience and their objectives. Other necessary education is available through professional societies, graduate schools, information technology vendors, and consulting groups. The health care institution should financially support employee efforts to take advantage of these opportunities for learning. Team members can also brush up on specific technology by visiting other institutions to observe the information technology in action.

Understanding Institutional Processes

Specific activities can also be planned to help project team members better understand the hospital's institutional processes that the new system will affect. Well-managed learning activities not only contribute to the project's success, but also cause important collective learning and growth throughout the institution.[18]

Training and learning have one more important effect on project team members. Researchers have determined that recent management-related training of any kind induces positive and motivating perceptions of computer technology's potential benefits.[19]

Contracting for Outside Assistance

An implementation project often requires the expertise of professionals who are not cost justified by the institution's continuing operations. When such skills and knowledge are necessary, outside experts can be engaged for assistance.

One frequently chosen option is to contract for services from the firm marketing the selected information system. Vendor representatives are more knowledgeable about their own technology than other firms are likely to be, and they are often able to provide help in planning and implementing system modifications. They also usually contribute other invaluable technical assistance during system implementation.

In other cases, however, independent consultants may be more useful. Vendor representatives frequently have a narrow perspective on the range of alternatives available to decision makers; independent consultants can be more objective in selecting among technology options and management alternatives involving other vendors' products. Consequently, independent consultants may be more effective both at considering technology options and at offering critical and unbiased evaluations. For example, vendor representatives may suppress information about flaws or problems in their company's product or service, leaving those problems unaddressed and possibly unsolved. On the other hand, independent consultants have no reason to hide such details.

At several points in the implementation project, complex technical issues could arise that require assistance from extremely specialized experts. Successful use of local area networking and advanced telecommunications connections, for instance, requires that a myriad of detailed specifications be declared, using technical language decipherable only by the people who work in this field daily. Experts can be engaged either to help plan these details or to review details that have been specified by the system vendor or project team members.

It is also useful to call occasionally for outside review of major project decisions or of project status and plans at major milestones. These periodic reviews by outside experts could offer project team participants the advantage of a fresh look. Such a review might take the form of a one-day summary status meeting during which an outside expert asks questions, possibly challenges critical decisions, and offers suggestions. Even when such meetings reveal no problems, expectations of a periodic review process force the project manager and project team to examine their activities through the eyes of an objective outside expert engaged to critique the project.

Installing the System

Site Preparation

Projects that include acquisition of new computer hardware and additional video terminals also usually involve physical changes to the facility. Implementation may require preparation of space for equipment, installation of electrical power and air-conditioning, telecommunications arrangements with local telephone companies, and cabling or networking to interconnect equipment or to connect terminals to computers. And when new computer equipment is installed, it's also prudent to put in place special control and alarm systems for water detection, smoke detection, fire detection and suppression, and monitoring and controlling physical access to the computer equipment area.

While the system vendor may provide site preparation assistance in support of new system installation, management may also want to consider local architectural and contracting firms as alternative suppliers of these services. Competitive bidding among such firms could generate lower costs than those proposed by the system vendor.

Computer Hardware and Software

After site preparations are completed, installation of vendor products begins. First, computer hardware, computer terminal equipment, and telecommunications and networking equipment are installed. The vendor's software product, often called the *base version* of the software, is then installed. Identifying this software with a version number or other label helps differentiate it from both previous and subsequent versions, which may include different functions and may or may not include the latest corrections to reported errors. It's also wise to test and validate the software to ensure that the installed base version is the correct version, with the capabilities and functions described in the vendor proposal.

Installing the base version of vendor software in a special software repository allows it to be easily monitored and controlled. All computer systems store computer programs internally in software repositories, sometimes called *software libraries,* from which the programs are automatically retrieved when scheduled or otherwise requested. The repository in which the base version is loaded should be identified as such, and the software should also be loaded or copied into another, separate repository. Managerial controls can then be imposed to ensure that authorized software changes and modifications are made only to the second repository, thus protecting the base version for later use as a reference. As software corrections and customization take place, various copies of customized computer programs frequently evolve, and it could be useful to access the original base version as an aid during problem solving. When a future version of the vendor's software become available, comparing it with the earlier base version helps pinpoint changes to any computer program in the new version.

During installation, the vendor should be required to deliver several copies of an instruction manual that includes both technical reference material for use in managing and maintaining the computer processing, and instructional reference material for end users of the system. Again, identifying this documentation with a version number helps differentiate it from other versions and links it with the corresponding software. The health care institution should designate an employee to serve as librarian. Most vendors have some organized method of distributing updated documentation, and management can request that any new information be mailed to the librarian, who then distributes the updates to documentation holders throughout the institution.

Customization and Integration

An institution implementing comprehensive information systems chooses from a vast and exponentially growing array of information technology options. Some of these options are considered and chosen during the system acquisition process, while defining requirements and selecting a vendor proposal. However, many options are still available for consideration during system implementation. Moreover, the system's ultimate value to the institution may depend more on customization options chosen during implementation than on any decisions made during the acquisition process.

Considering institutional characteristics

Reimbursement regulations or contractual obligations create the need for some customization enhancements. Other enhancements are necessary simply because the institution offers some special service, such as patient transportation via helicopter, or has some special management interest, such as detailed record keeping for outpatient encounters.

A truly successful information system provides features that are tailored to the work of the institution. Institutions that completely force-fit their work to a vendor's product are essentially handicapping their own systems, because the full realization of benefits from an benefits information system depends on how well its capabilities fit the institution. As studies indicate: "The more adaptable a system to different managers and different needs, the better the fit. . . . The better the fit of a system to a manager's cognitive style, the greater the likelihood that the manager will use it."[20]

Customization can be used effectively to tailor a system to the institution's unique culture and management style. Level of detail and degree of data summarization in printed reports, for example, can be customized, just as software for patient billing and collections can be made to conform with the institution's management methods and strategies. Controls on data security, controls on management of changes to the institution's computerized charge description manual, and rigidity of controls on what data must be entered as part of a registration can also be customized to fit the institution's needs.

The system can additionally be molded to meet internal technological conventions and standards. Such items as screen formats and networking protocols can be customized for consistency with those of related systems to prevent confusion among users about differing terminology and keyboard conventions.

Furthermore, the best system is one that is flexible for evolving institutional culture and adaptable for future customizing. As users gain experience with the system, they become better equipped to specify enhancements that will improve the system's fit to the institution. It is with a continually improving fit that the real benefits of a new information system are realized. The more flexible and adaptable the system is to this continued customization, the greater its likelihood of success.

Continued customization is a complex task requiring technical competence and careful management, however, because enhancements may introduce risk of error or make usage more difficult to manage. Customization could cause software, for example, to function in a manner previously untested, exposing the institution to yet undetected errors. Complex enhancements could also make error diagnosis and correction extremely difficult. Moreover, enhancements may complicate installation of future upgrades to vendor software.

Organizing work

Implementation of a new computer system is much more likely to succeed if work management and information flow problems of the departments of the institution are first identified and resolved. A computer system that simply automates unorganized work is doomed to fail, just as the manual processes preceding it failed.[21] Poorly organized departments experiencing work management problems may mistakenly seek computer automation as a solution to their problems, either naively grasping for a solution or deviously trying to divert attention from the real problems.

Here again, the project team helps provide a solution. Project team members also represent departments on the periphery of the work to be automated, not just the department that will be principally affected by the new system. Working together, these representatives can propose enhancements to work flow that improve its efficiency or usefulness for their departments. Such proposals inevitably raise questions about a department's poorly organized work and lead to its reorganization.

Customizing with prototyping

Some of the implementation project's most sensitive and critical work focuses on defining the precise details of work to be performed by users at video terminals. This definition activity, involving what are often called *human factors*, includes specifying data to be displayed on screens, formats and sequence of screens, required keyboard entry by users working at terminals, and system responses when users perform their work correctly or incorrectly. Users' perceptions and acceptance of the entire system hinge on how well they understand and accept these details.

For this reason, prototyping is extremely effective during the definition of video screen formats. Prototype versions of the screens may be created, reviewed by users, and then refined gradually and repeatedly until users accept them. A prototype version of a video screen usually includes only screen format and content, not all logic and processing that takes place behind the scenes. Consequently, it typically takes only a matter of hours to prepare or change the prototype version. A prototyping approach gives users the opportunity to contribute directly, helping define the work that they will perform at their terminals and also giving them a feeling of participation, both of which improve the project's chances of success.

Prototyping may also be used just as effectively to choose among options when defining the format and content of computer-printed reports. Decisions must be made about the placement of columns on pages, wording of page headings, wording of column headings, sequence of data on the pages, and other details that highlight the important items on reports. Prototype versions may be defined and distributed to potential users, then continually refined until the details are most useful and acceptable.

Customizing with profiles and tables

In anticipation of customers' needs, software vendors design their products to accommodate some customization. Software often includes features that allow institutions to declare their choices among system options.

These options are usually entered into the system in the form of changes to tables or profiles, which are stored in the computer system as reference lists that the system retrieves and invokes as it performs processing. For example, special codes identifying different types of patients' insurance coverage may be stored in such a table, as might the wording of the several alternative phrases to be printed on statements of overdue accounts. Many other details are specified using tables and profiles: format of pharmacy medication and laboratory specimen labels, the names of hospital departments, the names and cost centers of nursing stations, names of buildings, and names of the corporate entities of the institution. Tables and profiles may additionally define diverse control parameters, such as the minimum data required to perform a patient registration, criteria for selecting patient accounting data to archive, how long data should be archived before being purged, and length of time that a password is valid.

Similarly, specifications for video screen content and format are usually declared in the form of near-images of the video screens, which are then stored in special libraries for retrieval and use by the system as it performs processing. For example, an image is declared of the video screen containing wording and specific instructions for users who are signing on. That image is entered into the system, where it is stored in a special library. Then, when a user attempts to sign on to the system, the system retrieves the stored image, merges it with other data (such as the date and time), and presents the end product at the user's video terminal.

Tables and profiles are also used to declare the format and content of printed reports. Report titles, columns, instructions for sorting and ranking data on reports, and columnar arithmetic may be declared, stored, and then invoked by the system when the reports are scheduled for processing.

Customizing with computer programming

Although some items can be customized through declarations that are entered into tables and profiles, other adjustments require computer programming. The institution may need additional reports, for example, that the vendor's product doesn't include. Or modest changes may be necessary to facilitate data exchange between the new system and an already installed system that uses additional or different data fields. Complex computer programming changes can additionally provide system functions required by special business needs, such as including special patient classifications required by the state or regional peer review organization (PRO), or providing special productivity enhancements that potentially reduce patients' length of stay.

Computer programming is a multistep process that provides specific instructions for a computer to follow. The computer programming work, performed by computer programmers, begins with a design step defining both what the computer program is to do and the precise logic for how it is to do it, including specification of arithmetic formulas, if applicable. The actual computer programming, or *coding*, then begins, resulting in one or more sets of computer instructions, or programs. A clear and thorough design is crucial: it helps a computer programmer produce a structured and orderly program just as a good outline helps a writer compose complete and logical text. Good design additionally allows easy delegation of computer programming work among several computer programmers—and possibly into several separate computer programs. Finally, a detailed and orderly computer program is much easier to later read and review, aiding in future error diagnosis and installation of further customization enhancements.

After computer programming is complete, the resulting computer programs are tested to determine if they perform the required functions logically and correctly. During the testing process, errors are diagnosed, corrections to computer programs are made, and the programs are retested. This cycle, called *debugging*, is designed to eliminate all *bugs* from the programs: it is repeated until no additional errors are uncovered. Unfortunately, not all combinations of data and conditions can be simulated in a testing environment. Errors that are left undetected may cause system failure after the programs are placed in use, requiring diagnosis and correction at that later time.

In some cases, customization requires that new and additional computer programs be written; in other cases, modifications must be made to computer programs provided by the vendor. Modifications to computer programs are more difficult and riskier than new programs because changes may cause malfunction of the vendor's software, making error diagnosis more difficult and also possibly invalidating the vendor's warranty or maintenance support contract. Moreover, only careful documentation of all modifications can maintain compatibility with subsequent versions of vendor software. For example, when the vendor provides future versions of computer programs, each updated computer program must be analyzed to determine if it was previously modified. A significant amount of intellectual work may then be necessary to design an equivalent modification for the new version.

Transition to First Use

Switchover—sometimes also called *cutover* or *conversion*—is the critical transition during which the new system and procedures replace manual or old systems and procedures. During this period, management plays a vital role. Many tightly scheduled activities are highly dependent on each other; many important decisions will be made. The transition process also usually reaches a point of no return, and the decision at that juncture to go forward or not could have dramatic—or drastic—impact. In short, a poorly managed transition could create a major crisis for the institution.

Three basic techniques are available for making the actual change from the old systems and procedures to the new. Two methods prescribe a phased process; the third, called *crash switchover,* involves substituting the entire new system for the old in one step. A crash switchover puts both the project and the institution at great risk and should be avoided unless no other technique is feasible.

One phasing technique, called *pilot switchover* or *phased switchover,* involves allowing the system to be used by a small part of the institution for a short time, during which unfamiliar processes and potential problems are experienced. System use is then expanded to a larger group, a larger set of functions, or both. For example, one nursing station may use a new order entry function for a while before its use is extended to other nursing units. Or a new billing system may first be used only on outpatient billing for a period, then extended to inpatient billing.

Another phasing technique, *parallel operation,* involves operating both the old and the new system simultaneously and in parallel with each other until the new system is deemed to be performing properly. For example, patient charge processing may be performed by both old and new processes, and the results of each closely monitored. When both processes give equivalent results, then the old process is discontinued and switchover to the new process is consummated.

Organizational Changes

As new systems and procedures are defined, training begins, and employees become familiar with new procedures, personnel and organizational behavior problems inevitably surface. During transition, group attitudes have their greatest influence on the system's ultimate success, possibly even limiting expected benefits.

Clinical personnel especially may be wary and negative, since the change may be threatening and stressful to them. Researchers have concluded that professional people who have little past exposure to information technology have inaccurate perceptions and negative attitudes,[22] and this condition must be overcome if the system implementation is to be successful.

Throughout this period, management can counter negative factors by identifying key supervisors, managers, physicians, and other influential group leaders, convincing them of the system's benefits, negotiating with them, and persuading them to support it. Their aid is also vital for recognizing and dealing with informal coalitions among employees or physicians. As soon as distinct groups are identified that may resist computer processes or change in general, communication and training can be fashioned to improve their perception of the systems and procedures being implemented.[23]

Transition is also a time when management can help ensure the system's success by maintaining constant vigilance for organizational problems that could occur as the switchover from old responsibilities to new responsibilities begins. Specifically, great stress may be placed on lower-level supervisors and managers, who could feel threatened by organizational shifts in power and begin to resist change.[24] The more sensitive and adaptable management is to these organizational change issues, the lower the likelihood of conflict, resistance, and implementation difficulty.[25]

In addition to institutionwide changes, organizational changes will also take place within information services departments. Major responsibilities of the applications support departments decline, while new responsibilities begin for the computer production services departments.

Communicating with Users

The project team can reduce resistance to use of new systems and procedures by communicating with users and encouraging their commitment to successful use of the new system. Researchers have determined that good communication between users and implementers effectively lowers conflict levels.[26] Information about possible reorganization and changes in job responsibilities is especially important for reducing apprehension and stress. It's vital to positively influence as many potential users as possible because preventing users' perceptions of power loss also prevents conflict.[27]

Communication with physicians is becoming increasingly important as physicians are more involved and affected by new information systems. Some physicians may be ready and willing to accept more automation in patient care, but others are less convinced, possibly doubtful, of computer systems' usefulness, making the implementation process very dependent on the success of communication processes with physicians.

The best method for achieving these goals begins with documentation that is designed specifically for each intended audience, using both paper and electronic media. Paper reference manuals must be available to information services professionals; paper instruction manuals should be available to users. Video screens can be programmed to provide quick references and general instructions so that users at their terminals can directly access the system for timely and easy answers to inquiries, such as the proper insurance codes to use, or for explanations of brief error messages.

Project team members are uniquely qualified to assume responsibility for communicating as broadly as necessary to potentially affected users throughout the health care institution. For example, departmental liaison representatives should schedule departmental start-up activities, resolve problems, coordinate assignment of user passwords, and handle related data security issues. Other project team members can discuss relevant implementation topics at meetings of management, nurses, and physicians.

The information services organization is also well equipped to bear responsibility for communicating to users. The help desk, for example, serves as the primary source of assistance and information for terminal users. Help desk employees who are provided with appropriate information to communicate are in an ideal position to disseminate it. The help desk can also be given responsibility for electronically sending periodic messages to all users. Distributing a periodic newsletter is also an effective strategy for enhancing effective communication with users.

Training

Switchover to a comprehensive new information system means training large numbers of employees in many departments and in many different skills. Personnel in computer operations, production control, data security administration, and other information services areas will also undergo training. Users who perform functions at video screens will also require training, as will users who handle other daily transactions involving the new system. Management and supervisory people who schedule work need to be familiar with the new system's specific capabilities and ready to use them for work management. Specific gatekeeper positions will be defined to ensure that certain system transactions, such as changes to charge codes, receive appropriate approvals at appropriate authority levels; employees assigned to these positions will require training.

The phasing and timing of training are important. Trainers, liaison people, and supervisory people will naturally be trained first. Supervisors who are trained before their staffs can answer questions as employees ask them. Also, having been trained first, supervisors will be perceived as more knowledgeable, which in turn will help them both to support the changes that the system is bringing and to successfully encourage staff acceptance of the changes.

Switchover to the new computer information system cannot take place until an adequate number of employees are trained to perform critical required skills on all shifts, including weekends. Again, timing for training is critical: it can't start before the training version of the system is functional, but it must begin early enough to allow time for training the number of potential users necessary for switchover to occur. Writing an outline of skills needed, by phase of installation, helps the project team to plan effectively the sequence in which training should be scheduled and decide how to package and schedule training modules over a period of time.

Training designed to develop skills in using system capabilities ideally takes place directly at computer terminals, and students who receive individual attention as they are exercised and tested learn more quickly. The best training site, therefore, is a computer training center containing a small number of terminals and utilizing a training version of the system being installed. A training version functions exactly as the real system does, but it allows access to fictional patients of fictional institutions. This protects real patients' confidential data and hospital operations while also allowing students to enter fictional data and make mistakes.

To ensure that only qualified employees use the new system, minimum proficiency standards should be established, and any students who cannot meet them should be screened out. In most cases, the personnel scheduled for training are those who currently perform the equivalent work using current systems and procedures. But many of these people may be unqualified even for the jobs they perform, having never before been subject to screening for minimum qualifications. Therefore, training sessions and assessments may actually impose minimum job qualifications for the first time—and some employees may not meet minimum skill requirements. In such cases, reassignment of these employees requires careful management attention and could become a sensitive issue.

Once training is complete, and the system switchover is scheduled and completed, continued training and in-services are required to train future new hires and as a refresher for those who may require it.

Data Conversion

Existing data records must be prepared for first use in the new system. This process begins by assigning a project team member to determine which data records can be prepared by copying them directly from the old computerized records. Some additional data records may be prepared by transforming old data records to new data requirements using logic (that is, translating old codes to new codes). Computer programs are needed for both types of conversion. The new system might also require new data that are not available from the old system; these data must be collected and entered manually.

Although some data can be converted in advance, most data are changing right up to the point of the switchover. Dynamic factors such as patient location and patient orders, for example, place data conversion activity on the critical path of the switchover. There is no alternative but to convert this kind of data at the actual point of the switchover, after the old system is stopped and before the new system is started.

Testing and System Acceptance

Other switchover preparations focus on thorough testing of all system capabilities with the prescribed input data to determine if they function correctly and generate the proper output. A complete test plan ensures not only that tests of all capabilities are specifically assigned to individuals, but also that capabilities are sequentially tested to cover all dependencies. When testing patient registration processing, for example, testing data input capabilities first confirms that the proper data enter the system and are stored correctly; face sheet processing and other output can then be tested to ensure that stored data are properly utilized.

The best approach is simple and methodical: all data entry is tested, and all reports are printed and validated. Data input testing with both correct and incorrect data ensures that correct data are properly accepted while incorrect data are properly rejected. Testing should also validate processing through all data cycles, through all integrated functions and interfaces, and during daily or other periodic start-up and shut-down. Finally, it's vital to test all the user requirements stated in the RFP and vendor proposal. This ensures that the system actually meets all requirements, with no capabilities left missing or untried.

Such a rigorous effort is best accomplished by assigning specific testing and validation of results to project team members and to other employees, managers, and, potentially, physicians outside the project team. Including these outsiders in the testing process not only increases the number of people available for testing, but also improves potential users' acceptance of the system because they contribute to its implementation.

The latter steps of system testing usually lead to parallel operation, during which the new system temporarily functions in harmony with old systems and procedures, under normal loads and under special higher-than-normal loading, through all major data cycles. The results of both processes are compared to ensure that they are equivalent. Also during parallel operation, processing loads and on-line response times are measured and closely checked against expectations and contractual specifications.

Successful completion of testing and parallel operation is a major milestone in the implementation project. And assessment of the testing results is critical, since acceptance usually leads to the point of no return. When the project manager or other designated management person declares the parallel operation to be successful enough that the new system should continue processing and the old system should be discontinued, a return to the old system is usually impossible even if difficulties are later uncovered. At this point, a system acceptance milestone is usually assumed unless some exceptions are noted among vendor and customer representatives. As major acceptance milestones are successfully reached, corresponding payments are then made to the vendor.

Problem Management

Problem management is one of the project manager's primary responsibilities during the testing process, throughout parallel operation and acceptance, and especially after passing the point of no return, when the institution can no longer revert to the safety afforded by the old system. Problem-reporting procedures and forms (as shown in Exhibit 3.4 and described in Chapter 3) that are carefully defined and used by all participants can help ensure that all problems are addressed. Methods for tracking problem resolution can also be put in place to ensure that the highest-priority problems are being addressed, to verify that qualified people are assigned to resolve problems, to document that all participants know of any problem's occurrence and impact, and to clarify vendor responsibilities and responsiveness in solving problems during these critical periods. In some cases, the problem-reporting methods must conform to provisions of the vendor's contract, which may require that problems be reported using some defined format or process or within some defined time period. For example, the vendor's contract may state that problems must be reported to a specific vendor representative, using a special form, and within a specific number of hours after occurrence.

Hazards and Contingency Plans

Even with the most competent management and thorough plans, the testing and system acceptance process is fraught with difficulties, and the project manager faces many critical decisions about continuing—or discontinuing and rescheduling—the processes. Converted data may be discovered to be incomplete or incompatible. Computer programs may fail. Incorrect versions of data or computer programs may be improperly loaded into software libraries. Someone may incorrectly perform conversion tasks so that the wrong version of data is put into use. Such hazards call for management procedures that ensure that problems are reported and recorded, consequences of problems are assessed, and problem resolution activities are prioritized and addressed quickly. Only such procedures can arm the project manager for assessing problems and their consequences and deciding among options.

As problems are faced during system implementations, executive management must ensure that project managers constantly assess available options and the accompanying exposure to risk—and both options and risks change dramatically after the point of no return is passed. Up to this point, it may be possible to restore old files and programs and revert to old systems and procedures. Even after passing the point of no return, there may be options to suspend processing temporarily while some major problem is addressed. With some dynamic patient record-keeping processes, such as patient registration, however, even a brief pause may not be feasible. In such cases, shifting to a manual record-keeping process, using a form similar to that shown in Exhibit 7.2, may be a short-term alternative—that is, if such a manual process, including appropriate forms, procedures, and training, has been previously provided. Another option in the face of problems is to reduce the scope of the effort, proceeding with some parts of the system while deferring others. Furthermore, as problems are uncovered, resolved, and the system restarted, it may sometimes be plausible first to restore files and programs as they were at an earlier step in the process, and then direct users to revert back and repeat their work from that point. Procedures for auto-

will be described in Chapter 8.

The project manager can never place too much importance on the critical event marking the point after which return to old systems and procedures is no longer possible. Specifically, it may be wise to cross that point only after a brief meeting where project team members reach consensus about making the decision. In no case should vendor representatives be allowed to make this crucial decision; because the vendor's payment may be linked to this milestone, its representatives could be tempted to inappropriately expose the customer to great risk in the interest of the vendor's financial benefit.

Change Management

During any implementation project, system changes will inevitably be made. As project team members and other participants become familiar with system capabilities, they often propose enhancements. During testing, parallel processing, and system acceptance activities, latent system flaws emerge and require system modifications.

One method to manage these changes effectively and minimize the accompanying risk is change management: All proposals for system enhancements are defined on a form designed specifically for that purpose,

Exhibit 7.2 Sample Form for Manual Recording During Computer Downtime

---

Downtime Form   **Control No: 36846**

This form is to be used only when the HIS is down. When the computer is again operating, it is the responsibility of the department with the white copy to enter the transaction into the system.

Patient account: 0123456-1289   Nursing unit: M7SE

Patient name: Smith, Jane   Date: 12/16/89   Time: 10:15 p.m.

Patient room/bed: M708B   Entered by: Nancy Brown

                                       Extension: x6175

Ordered by: Dr. John Doe, M.D.

Transaction/order: P.T. Consult - ORTHO

---

explaining both the enhancements and their justification. During implementation, project team members review these proposals and approve justified enhancements if they are feasible and do not add unnecessary risk to the project.

Each change, whether it results from proposed enhancements or as a solution to problems, is documented, programmed if necessary, installed, and tracked to ensure that it functions correctly. When the change involves revising or adding a new computer program, the change should be declared on a special form (such as that shown in Exhibit 3.2 and described in Chapter 3) listing both a reference to the source of the change's requirement and such details as the name of the computer program being changed or newly created, the version number of the prior and new program versions, the persons performing the work, details of testing, relevant dates and times, and the approval signature of the responsible manager. When the change requires revision of a reference table or profile, a similar form (Exhibit 7.3) is used to declare the intent, provide information about the change, and gain the responsible manager's signature. Data from forms of both types are then consolidated into one list and presented as the agenda of periodic change management meetings, where managers and technical personnel approve or reject the proposed changes and their schedules for implementation.

Change management procedures also apply when vendors periodically issue new versions of a system, involving new versions of all or many of the computer programs that make up the system. The vendor may additionally provide interim computer program changes as remedies for reported system problems. Receipt, installation, and testing of these interim program changes can also be effectively managed through prescribed change management procedures.

Postimplementation Activities

Preserving the Project Team

Even after the testing and acceptance processes are completed, the project team is kept intact to provide continuing support for users who experience difficulties and problems arising from changed work processes. It is vital that users have immediate access to help from members of the project team during the critical period following implementation, so that problems can be resolved quickly and behavior and attitude problems can be sensed and remedied quickly. The project team agenda during this period shifts to a

Exhibit 7.3 Sample Profile Change Form for Recording and Approving
Changes to Internal System Profiles and Tables

Requestor:	Jane Doe	Date: 12/4/89
Profile affected:	Demographic codes profile	
Reason for change:	Add new codes for observation patients, gender,	
	and financial class	

Type of Code	Code	Description/Details
Patient type	I	Inpatient
	O	Outpatient
	D	Day surgery
	V	Observation patient
Gender	F	Female
	M	Male
	U	Unspecified
Financial class	M	Medicare
	B	Blue Cross
	C	Commercial
	X	Medicaid
	S	Self-pay

heavy concentration on tracking problems, assessing system operation, and coordinating efforts to resolve problems and make other necessary changes.

Continued Surveillance

During the early postimplementation period, the principal activity focuses on closely monitoring system operations and providing responsive remedies to problems. Project team members assess system operation continuously to distinguish among system problems and personnel problems.

Work processes in all departments are reviewed and compared with expectations and planned changes. Problems of either work overloads or underutilization of employees are addressed. Worker competency is assessed, with additional training scheduled when necessary. If workers resist use of the system, new procedures and other management intervention are then defined to eliminate the cause of their resistance.

Special care is taken to assess work processes in departments where implementation of the new system has generated significant changes. Workers in these departments may decide the system imposes work processes that are too rigid and controlled and that do not provide options for handling important exceptions. For example, work procedures in some diagnostic departments are different on weekends when the departments have a skeleton staff, and weekday work management procedures may prevent the weekend staff from performing their work. System changes may be necessary to accommodate unforeseen requirements in such cases.

The postimplementation project team should also attempt to locate work processes that continue the parallel operation of both the old and new systems well after the automated processes have been fully tested and validated. Clinical personnel, for example, may not trust the new automated systems and procedures and may continue to perform the duplicate work of the old systems and procedures.

Careful assessment of work processes additionally uncovers any other issue that is causing negative impressions, although no system malfunction may be apparent. For example, the credibility of some process or system output may be in doubt. In such a situation, even when system errors have not surfaced, validation of the suspected process and data eliminates any suspicion.

Finally, work processes are assessed to determine if additional system controls are needed. For example, if data quality is eroded because incorrect data are entered into the system, additional or more rigid data edits may be considered. If user errors at one workstation are causing problems in other departments, added record keeping could pinpoint users who are making the mistakes.

As assessment progresses and potential enhancements are identified and justified, they are recorded, discussed within the project team, and prioritized. With the steering committee's approval, some enhancements are given high priority and implemented immediately to remedy difficulties in work processes and add necessary controls. These selected enhancements are then installed under the close guidance of the project team.

Problem management and performance monitoring also continue during the postimplementation period. Problems are reported, recorded, prioritized, and assigned. System performance is constantly monitored to ensure continued performance as specified in the formal documents of the RFP and vendor proposal.

Additionally, vendor service is carefully assessed, since the vendor may have reassigned its original installation staff to another client. Furthermore, a vendor that has received all payments may have little financial incentive to be as attentive as necessary.

To ensure that subtleties of new operations are clearly defined and well understood, work processes in the information services departments are also assessed. The computer production services department assumes appropriate responsibility for successfully operating the system as project team activities decline. For example, only help desk employees who thoroughly understand the new system can efficiently respond to users' problems. Likewise, the application systems departments assume responsibilities that were formerly borne by the project team. When the vendor later distributes magnetic tapes and user documentation containing software corrections or major updates to software, the corrections or updates are carefully analyzed and scheduled for installation. After analysis, some may appear to be optional. These corrections and updates should still be installed, however, no matter how dubious their benefit because subsequent versions may require that these earlier ones be in place before they can be used with their complete capabilities.

Also during the postimplementation period, the system's operational costs are compared against budgeted costs to determine any costs beyond those expected. Some vendor service expenses may exceed those proposed in the budget, for example, due to misunderstandings in the vendor's billing offices, and those misunderstandings and errors should be corrected.

Finally, several months after the acceptance and first use of the system, it is often helpful to administer a user survey. Questions about the system's capabilities, its usefulness, users' skill and familiarity with the system, and the support that they receive when problems occur can yield valuable insights. These insights help to perpetually enhance the system so that it evolves to provide advantages that the steering committee anticipated when it originally approved the project.

Notes

1. L. W. DiGuilio and T. K. Zinn, "Actualizing System Benefits—Part III," *Computers in Healthcare* (July 1988): 26–28.
2. J. G. Anderson et al., "Physician Use of HIS Impacts Quality of Care," *U.S. Healthcare* (October 1989): 41–42, 46.
3. A. G. Watlington, "Realizing System Benefits: Meeting the Implementation Challenges," *Computers in Healthcare* (May 1989): 28–29, 31–33.
4. A. G. Watlington, "Benefits Realization at Mercy Memorial Results in a Changed Organizational Culture," *Computers in Healthcare* (August 1989): 26–29, 32.

5. B. Minard, "Growth and Change Through Information Management," *Hospital & Health Services Administration* 32, no. 3 (August 1987): 307–18.
6. P. Federico, *Management Information Systems and Organizational Behavior* (New York: Praeger Publishers, 1985), p. 14.
7. P. Ein-Dor and E. Segev, *A Paradigm for Management Information Systems* (New York: Praeger Publishers, 1981), p. 148.
8. Ibid., p. 209.
9. G. J. Mann, "Managers, Groups, and People: Some Considerations in Information System Change," *Health Care Management Review* 14, no. 4 (Fall 1988): 43–48.
10. Ein-Dor and Segev, *A Paradigm*, p. 153.
11. Ibid., pp. 199, 206.
12. Ibid., p. 180.
13. Ibid., p. 209.
14. D. W. Young, "What Makes Doctors Use Computers," in *Use and Impact of Computers in Clinical Medicine*, ed. J. G. Anderson and S. J. Jay (New York: Springer-Verlag, 1987), pp. 8–14.
15. D. J. Mishelevich et al., "Implementation of the IBM Health Care Support/Patient Care System," in *Information Systems for Patient Care*, ed. B. I. Blum (New York: Springer-Verlag, 1984), pp. 62–82.
16. J. G Anderson and S. J. Jay, "The Diffusion of Computer Applications in Medical Settings," in *Use and Impact of Computers in Clinical Medicine*, ed. J. G. Anderson and S. J. Jay (New York: Springer-Verlag, 1987), pp. 3–7.
17. Ein-Dor and Segev, *A Paradigm*, pp. 208–9.
18. Minard, "Growth and Change."
19. Ein-Dor and Segev, *A Paradigm*, pp. 208–9.
20. Ibid., p. 211.
21. DiGuilio and Zinn, "Actualizing System Benefits."
22. E. Zoltan-Ford and A. Chapanis, "What Do Professional Persons Think About Computers?" in *Use and Impact of Computers in Clinical Medicine*, ed. J. G. Anderson and S. J. Jay (New York: Springer-Verlag, 1987), pp. 51–67.
23. Ein-Dor and Segev, *A Paradigm*, p. 191.
24. F. W. McFarlan and J. L. McKenney, *Corporate Information Systems Management: The Issues Facing Senior Executives* (Homewood, IL: Richard D. Irwin, Inc., 1983), p. 17.
25. Ein-Dor and Segev, *A Paradigm*, pp. 203–5.
26. Ibid., pp. 202–3.
27. Ibid.

8

PROTECTION AND CONTROLS FOR INFORMATION SYSTEMS ASSETS: DATA SECURITY, DATA INTEGRITY, AND DISASTER PREVENTION

The quality of a patient's medical care depends fundamentally on the reliability and accuracy of the hospital's computer information systems and on the quality of cumulative computerized records that are compiled and shared among clinical personnel who provide that care. For example, treatment depends on information such as age and allergies, recorded during the patient's registration, and depends also on the recorded results of laboratory tests.

Similarly, the hospital's efficient daily operation and profitability depend on accurate and timely recording of such information as services and tests ordered, patient location, patient charges, and payments received.

Furthermore, mismanagement of the hospital's information systems could cause major discontinuity or failure. To protect against such vulnerability, executive management bears the important responsibility for assessing risks and imposing appropriate controls that ensure the continuing successful operation of the hospital's computer systems.

The Need for Concern and Action

Recent headlines about insidious computer viruses in large governmental computer networks dramatize the widespread vulnerability of computer information systems. Furthermore, recently publicized security breaches in large computer information systems are eroding the public's confidence in such systems. Such concerns should evoke executives' anxieties about their own institution's exposure to malfunctioning computer systems.

Computer information systems, of course, cannot be expected to operate without some exposure to failure. Even the most well-designed information systems are subject to problems with data integrity and computer failure. People inevitably make errors when they use computer information systems. For many employees and physicians, their use of computers in the hospital may be their first experience with computers, and unfamiliarity often breeds mistakes. Moreover, the vast differences that exist among methods and conventions used in different computer systems frequently cause even experienced users to use commands and conventions in one system that are valid only in another system. Finally, the stressful work conditions that exist in many patient care areas (such as an emergency room or an ICU) create an atmosphere in which data-recording errors are likely to occur. To limit these considerable exposures to errors, however, specific countermeasures can be put in place. These countermeasures may be as simple as providing excellent training, or as complex as designing a system that has thorough error checking and detailed instructions for remedies to problems.

Management faces a diversity of interrelated problems in managing the protection of computer information system assets. Patient data must be kept confidential. Corporate information assets must be kept secure. Computer equipment and data files must be protected from destruction. People's confidence in computer information systems must be built and maintained. And, finally, the health care institution's employees and medical staff must accept the responsibilities of using this technology. In the face of these problems, executives must acknowledge the health care institution's potential exposure to risk of inoperable systems and data loss, with the resulting negative effect on operations, and they must impose the expectation that the best possible countermeasures against such exposures be devised.

Concentrated Computer Technology Assets

The computer equipment and data bases of information systems of a health care institution are usually concentrated in one location. This physical concentration exposes all these components to anyone attempting unauthorized access and therefore creates an increased security problem for the institution. For example, an unauthorized person could program a personal computer to dial all combinations of phone numbers until the personal computer identifies another computer system responding. The same person could then program the personal computer to connect with the identified computer system and systematically try many combinations of access passwords. If access is eventually gained, a short period of electronic access can provide data equivalent to that contained in many file cabinets of manual records. Once data are obtained, the computational power of a personal computer enables its operator to piece together and decipher data from several files, making the stolen information even more valuable. In a similar manner, unauthorized users can access computer systems to change stored data, corrupting or destroying information or even defrauding the health care institution.

Human error has a potent leveraged influence in computer information systems because one person's error can so quickly affect the work of others. One person's mistake, possibly by a computer operator, for example, could destroy the accuracy of data entered by personnel throughout the hospital, requiring whole departments to reenter data transactions. Likewise, mistakes made by custodians of major repositories of reference material, such as computer programs and manuals, could make that important material unuseable to others when they need it. Or someone's mistake with equipment in a wiring closet through which computer networks interconnect could ultimately fragment a computer network and render large segments inoperable. Catastrophic problems in a computer center, such as fire or water damage, could shut down a computer information system for a lengthy period.

The Causes of Unauthorized Information System Use

Attempts at unauthorized use of computer systems are usually rooted in one or more of three motivations: the challenge and personal thrill of breaking through formidable security barriers, the hostility of a disgruntled employee or other person critical of the institution, or the expectation of financial gain.

Computer enthusiasts who are challenged by, and receive a thrill from, breaking through data security protective barriers are called hackers. They can be outsiders who attempt to penetrate security over telephone lines, or they can be employees who try to exceed their authorization limits.

A hostile employee, vendor, customer, or other person, bitter over some disappointment, may vindictively attempt to sabotage or corrupt information in computerized data bases. Such an individual also may attempt to discredit the institution by retrieving confidential data, such as patient information, and passing the data on to the news media.

An unauthorized user seeking financial gain could defraud an institution by changing patient accounts, accounts payable records, or employee payroll records. Or data could be stolen and sold or otherwise used for financial gain. Patients' accounts data, for example, could be used to obtain fraudulent credit cards. Intellectual property, such as copies of computer programs, or physical property, such as personal computer equipment and supplies, also could be stolen and sold.

Confidentiality of Data: A Double-Edged Sword

To be useful, data must be easily available to health care workers who must have access to relevant information about medical tests and state of illness, both to administer care and to protect themselves from contagion. At the same time, however, each patient has a right to expect that personal data will be kept confidential, and the hospital is obligated to protect that confidential data from access by unauthorized parties.

Data confidentiality is much more than an abstract ideal; it is required by law. The wide use of computer information systems, beginning in the late 1960s, prompted widespread public concern over potential invasions of an individual's privacy. As a result, many federal laws (for example, the Freedom of Information Act of 1970, the Privacy Act of 1974, the Right to Financial Privacy Act of 1978, and the Comprehensive Crime Control Act of 1984) were enacted to protect privacy by establishing controls over the collection, storage, accuracy, and distribution of confidential data. Many state laws were patterned after these federal laws.

As health care information systems provide a growing amount of information to a more diverse and geographically distributed population of health care professionals, a new data security issue arises: the confidentiality of computerized records chronicling treatments administered, records that should not be reviewed for research or other purposes without specific authorization.

Consequently, to safeguard confidentiality, management should impose controls that prevent browsing and that guide each authorized user to the subset of relevant, authorized data.[1]

Intellectual Property: Protecting Software Rights

Another critical management issue centers on ownership of the intellectual property that new and valuable computer systems represent. The product of a health care institution's intellectual work has intrinsic value that should be acknowledged and protected. Such intellectual property, primarily in the form of computer programs, may be valuable to others. Another hospital could use it without repeating the owner's investment; a vendor could market it for others to purchase. Properly written institutional policies and regulations can protect against piracy of computer programs by employees, and properly written contracts can prevent vendors from obtaining and marketing software that the hospital should partially or exclusively own.

Risks: Threats and Exposures

We cannot expect computer information systems to operate free of errors and other exposures to failure, and we cannot expect people to work without making mistakes. But we can analyze why people make errors or, more specifically, how computer information systems allow such errors.

A great quantity of information has been published on security and controls in computer information systems. Unfortunately, much of this information is found in technical dissertations that fail to provide a practical framework for assessing risks and responding with countermeasures. To make matters worse, both terminology and theory are inconsistent in the literature.[2,3]

The brief set of terminology that follows, a composite of several published frameworks, offers a practical structure, identifying risks in such a way that countermeasures can be aimed specifically at each risk. In this composite, the business environment conditions outside the health care institution are identified as *causal agents*. These causal agents affect a health care institution at points of weakness, labeled *vulnerabilities*. Steps taken to limit the risks at these points of vulnerability are labeled *countermeasures*.

Causal Agents

Five causal agents exist in the working environment, several of which can appear either accidentally or as the result of an unauthorized intentional act.[4] These causal agents include the following:

1. People or procedures
2. Computer equipment
3. Computer software
4. Public utility services
5. Acts of nature

Vulnerabilities

Vulnerabilities are characteristic of a health care institution and its computer systems. For example, a hospital or its computer systems are vulnerable to flawed processes of collecting and entering data into computer systems, and processing of data in computer systems. The specific points of vulnerability listed here are an extension of material obtained from two primary sources.[5,6] These points of vulnerability are as follows:

1. Data collection: the possibility of errors (for example, transposition of numbers as they are entered on data entry forms), omissions, delays, and introduction of unauthorized data during data collection

2. Manual data input movement (for example, passing worksheets among people) and preparation of data for entry into the computer system: the possibility of data loss or modification and the introduction of unauthorized data during data movement

3. Data entry and communication of data to the computer: the possibility of errors (for example, keyboard mistakes), delays, omission of data, and the introduction of unauthorized data and software viruses as data enters the system

4. Data receipt, validation, and recording inside the computer: the possibility of insertion of data into an incorrect data cycle or system (for example, the computer operations department mistakenly processing a day's transactions twice)

5. Data processing in the computer: the possibility of computer malfunction and software malfunction (for example, flawed software)

6. Data output from the computer available only to authorized personnel: the possibility of confidential data being exposed to unauthorized people, the possibility of piracy of owned software and loss of intellectual property, and the possibility of piracy of vendor software

7. Data output movement for distribution to users: the possibility of loss or theft of magnetic tapes, microfiche, and reports as they are being distributed, and the possibility of others' interceptions of electronic data

8. Data receipt and usage by users: the possibility of loss or theft of magnetic tapes, microfiche, and reports from users' work areas

9. Data purging and archiving: the possibility of failure to properly dispose of data (for example, having confidential information intercepted from trash containers), the possibility of incorrectly destroying data that are still useful, and the possibility of inappropriately retaining data that are no longer necessary

Designing Computer Information Systems that Include Countermeasures

Computer information system countermeasures may be preventive, detective, or corrective. Each of these types of countermeasures will be discussed in the following sections.

Preventive Countermeasures

Preventive countermeasures limit unauthorized activity and guide authorized activity along a correct path. Such countermeasures however, are passive and usually offer no feedback on the frequency of a threat's occurrence. They are simply the first line of defense, reducing the probability and frequency of a threat.

Data quality assurance

Entering data into a computer information system is usually a tedious task and, therefore, a likely source of error. Data quality edits are preventive countermeasures that limit data entry errors. Such edits are quality assurance mechanisms that counter people's accidental or intentional activities.

One of the simplest data quality assurance measures involves providing detailed instructions for the collection of data and how it should be entered on forms, specifying what is required and what is optional, and under what conditions. Data collection worksheets that are organized to collect data in natural groupings result in a collection process that is more efficient and focused. Patient identification data can be organized for entry on one form, for example, while all insurance data are entered on another form, preventing illogical intermixing of information. Data can also be collected and prepared in natural cycles. For example, it is more logical to gather and prepare data daily than to save them for a week before organizing their preparation for entry into a computer system. This structure enables personnel performing the task, and possibly even the computer software, to sense errors such as the loss of an entire day's transactions.

Providing easy methods of data entry is another useful data quality assurance measure. A process of entering data by typing on keyboards is not only slow, it also has a high probability of error that reduces the credibility of results. An alternative method employing bar code readers and screen pointing devices can be used wherever possible to improve the accuracy of data entry processes. Data are also more accurate when data entry takes place at the first possible point of data collection, near the work of the transaction that is being recorded.

Computer software specifically designed for improving data quality can provide a means for imposing checks on the reasonableness of entered data. Such software is designed to be suspicious of errors most likely to be made, including transposition of digits in numeric data, such as patient numbers, quantities, and dates. Comprehensive computerized reasonableness checks include checking for valid dates, normal ranges of values, maximum or minimum quantities or dollars, correct patient numbers, and valid relationships among related data items such as birth date, sex, and service provided.

Data quality can also be safeguarded by ensuring that special codes used in computer systems are easy to learn and remember and are consistent and universal in different departments and computers throughout the hospital. For example, standard codes and abbreviations should exist for nursing stations and room numbering, for physician numbers and department numbers, and for all referral sources, third party payers, and local employers.

Use of standard forms is one more means of assuring data quality that is both simple to implement and effective. Easy-to-understand forms that include instructions and preprinted data reduce errors. Prenumbered forms can additionally prevent use of unauthorized substitute forms, as, for example, in the case of payroll or accounts payable checks. Also, the concept of a *turnaround document* limits errors. For example, a computer-printed document containing current employee data could be used to collect changed data, thereby eliminating any possibility of recording incorrect employee numbers as changes are made to other identifying or demographic data.

An additional measure for assuring data quality involves defining standard default values and standard procedures for handling exceptions. For example, all salaried people can be assumed to be working the normal 40 hours of a pay period unless an authorized exception is processed.

Authorization and approvals

Authorization is advance permission to initiate a transaction, and *approval* is the process of reviewing and allowing the transaction to proceed.[7] Both are preventive countermeasures, although approval is considered a detective countermeasure, and possibly even a corrective countermeasure, as well as a preventive countermeasure.

Authorization countermeasures not only govern access to computer system functions and data, but also govern manual processes such as access to blank checks. Approval countermeasures govern review, verification, and approval of data at key points before processing or data distribution can continue. For example, the accounting department's journal entries are usually approved before they are entered, and clinical lab data are usually verified and approved before they are printed or otherwise made available to physicians, nurses, and other clinical personnel.

Authorization and approval may also be intermixed. Such is the case when dual access control is imposed, requiring two people to be present or otherwise requiring two people to perform a function simultaneously. For example, two signatures could be required on certain checks, two keys could be necessary to enter some locked spaces, or two people could be required to be present to gain entry to certain areas.

Research protocols

Placing approval controls on access to patient data bases for research allows data to be used for valid research, while also ensuring data confidentiality. Medical staff and hospital management committee approval should be required before such data access is given, even if data are assumed to be "owned" by physicians on the service in which the data are collected.

Deliberate purging of data

The Privacy Act of 1974 addressed the public's growing concern that individual privacy might disappear altogether as computers collect more and more information about citizens. This and subsequent legislation provided controls on collection, dissemination, and use of data collected about individuals in our society. In particular, a growing body of legislation promotes the concept that data collected on individuals should have a finite life span. Each institution, therefore, needs some means of deciding which information is no longer useful, and that information should then be purged.

Physical security

Physical security plays an essential role in preventing access to certain locations, thereby keeping data and equipment assets secure. Offices where confidential data are collected and stored prior to entry into the computer should be locked after normal working hours. Confidential data being compiled should be kept in locked storage and, when mailed or sent to other departments, should be secured in packets marked and handled appropriately. Blank checks should also be stored in locked storage, and confidential output reports in secure office areas. Moreover, when printed documents containing confidential data are no longer useful, they should be destroyed by shredding or other controlled disposal.

Personal computers that store files of confidential data or other valuable institutional data should also be physically controlled. Such personal computers can be kept in locked offices or, alternatively, equipped with special locks that prevent operation without the key.

Passwords and variable menus

Passwords and user identification codes comprise a major preventive countermeasure by giving users access to limited subsets of computer functions and to limited subsets of data in an institution's data bases. The subset of functions and subset of data are typically controlled by specifying a menu of functions that the user first views after successfully signing on to the computer system. Users generally are allowed to change their passwords, but they can change neither their user identification codes nor the menu of functions available to them when they sign on. As an added countermeasure, users should be required to change their passwords periodically. Additionally, inactive user access codes and passwords should automatically be purged after a length of time slightly longer than one full processing cycle of the system, because a user who does not use the system during a full processing cycle, such as a month, may no longer be an active, authorized user. When a user makes a mistake in entering a password, the system should provide a limited number of retries before terminating the session. Then, if trial-and-error attempts continue, the system should automatically invalidate the user's access privilege and alert management of the need for follow-up, such as training the user or uncovering an attempt by a hacker.

Access control based on user access codes and associated variable menus lets users gain access to information they need while also limiting access to only necessary data. Granting access through passwords and variable menus provides the flexibility necessary to manage the trade-off between the need to make data easily available to caregivers and the need to keep data confidential.[8]

In utilizing this capability to provide flexible access, however, it may be tempting to produce what amounts to two-tiered security, methods of control that give higher concern to a special subset of data (such as VIP patients). This kind of strategy could eventually lead to legal difficulties: if data confidentiality problems arise, it could be shown that the more secure measures applied to VIPs could have been applied to all patients.

Ease of use

Another means of preventing errors is to make computerized work easy to perform and the system easy to use. Systems that are designed for ease of use are called *user friendly*.

In some computer information systems, messages and instructions displayed on video screens use indecipherable and confusing computer jargon that is too cryptic to be helpful. Confronted by such messages after having made simple mistakes, users do the best they can, but they nonetheless frequently make even worse mistakes, sometimes resulting in unpredictable and unrecoverable system errors. To prevent these problems, error messages should describe what is wrong and what the user should do. Moreover, for all video screen processes, the system should provide reversible processes. Consequently, when a user does make a mistake on such a system, the error can be corrected and the action can be undone, if necessary.[9]

The most effective messages and user conventions are consistent, understandable, and subject to enforced institutional standards. Users learn from continued use and, consequently, come to expect consistent terminology and conventions. Screen format can be designed so that instructions and information appear in the same place on all video screens, preventing users from making mistakes by incorrectly assuming consistent format and, consequently, making decisions based on the presence or absence of information in certain portions of the screen. Error messages, for example, should always appear in the same place on all video screens.[10]

Good fit of the system to need

Information technology defines or redefines the work of many people, and those responsible for this definition should recognize that system vulnerability to error will be determined largely by the attitudes and values of the people who ultimately work at the system's video terminals. When the system fits the health care institution's need, work is straightforward and workers gain a sense of work well done, both enhancing the meaningfulness of the work and the workers' motivation to perform it well. Workers' accountability for their work, and therefore its quality, will also be enhanced. On the other hand, if the system definition and design ignore these concepts—requiring users to bend the system and force it to do what it was not designed to do—the system may elicit contempt for both the work and its results, drastically increasing its vulnerability to problems.

Detective Countermeasures

Detective countermeasures provide a second line of defense against causal agents. They are designed to detect the presence of a causal agent that has penetrated a point of vulnerability. Ideally, detective countermeasures trigger some mechanism that brings about follow-up action to analyze and remedy the problem.[11]

Anticipation of scheduled outcome

A measure that tends to reduce data errors throughout the whole spectrum of data collection, data preparation, data entry, data processing, data output, and data distribution is the natural presence of an individual anticipating results from a scheduled activity. For example, employees expecting to receive a paycheck of a specified amount comprise one such countermeasure. Similarly, anticipation by department managers of certain levels of revenue is a natural detection measure. When effective natural detection measures are in place, other strong measures need not be imposed.

Computer reports

Computer reports provide one variation of the natural detection measure just described. In this approach, designated employees or managers receive computerized reports summarizing results of a computer processing cycle, such as the payroll cycle. They are then responsible for carefully reviewing the reports to determine reasonableness, missing data, and limits. The format of reports should present data in a sequence that highlights missing information, and the reports should also specifically list exceptions beyond norms, such as salaries or salary increases beyond a certain norm, departments with the most overtime, or departments with the greatest change in revenue during a specific time period.

Batch totals

In the type of computer processing known as batch processing, where transactions are collected for a period of time before processing takes place, use of *batch totals* is a detection measure imposed to ensure that all transactions have been processed once and only once. A clerk usually prepares a batch total by first calculating the sum of entries in a particular data field on all the documents and then entering that value in a batch control document that is entered into the computer together with the data. Subsequent comparison of totals calculated by the clerk with totals calculated by the computer potentially detects errors made during data preparation, data entry, and data processing.

Similarly, the computer can be made to calculate totals at each major step of a lengthy series of computer processing steps, called *run-to-run totals*. When these calculations are compared step to step, it ensures that the results of a previous computer processing step have not changed before the beginning of the next sequential step. Such a control guarantees that processing steps were not inadvertently skipped and that data were not lost as they passed from one processing step to the next.

Corrective Countermeasures

Corrective countermeasures automatically correct errors, directly specify what must be corrected, or assist in the correction of errors.

Reconciliation and matching

Reconciliation and matching is a corrective measure used to check two sets of data items that are expected to be similar, both to detect and to analyze differences between the two sets. For example, as we reconcile our personal bank statements each month, we determine which checks have not yet cleared and then either verify that our account balances are correct or uncover arithmetic errors and correct them.

In a variation on this process, another corrective measure allows reconciliation of results from two parallel and purposely redundant processes, verifying that matched results are accurate, and correcting results that do not match. When data entry processes employ this strategy, two data entry operators enter the same data, with the computer system alerting the second operator when entered data items do not match those entered by the first operator.

Equipment calibration

Because automated instruments are used in health care institutions to record data values and pass them into patients' data files, calibration of equipment is a major data quality concern. In these cases, sample data are periodically passed through the instruments, and the data results compared to the expected results. Differences are then calculated, and the results are used to recalibrate the instruments.

Periodic audits

An audit is a process of verifying that all countermeasures are being effectively applied to counter vulnerabilities. An audit may be performed by an internal auditor or by an auditor engaged from an auditing firm.

Periodic audits serve as a powerful countermeasure against all vulnerabilities by confirming that procedures are being properly performed and that data records are as expected. However, because an audit is also very time consuming and costly, it should be used only to determine the effectiveness of other countermeasures.

The Computer Utility and the Information Services Staff

This section focuses on countermeasures for departments within the information services organization, including the computer processing facility and its employees. Here again, countermeasures may be preventive, detective, or corrective.

Preventive Countermeasures

As stated earlier, preventive countermeasures serve as a first line of defense, limiting unauthorized activity and guiding authorized activity along a correct path.

Personnel countermeasures

Personnel countermeasures protect against people threats, and they are usually used to identify those employees who are authorized or responsible for certain activities. For example, job descriptions should state who is authorized to operate the computer and what levels of approval are required to stop and start the computer. Computer center instructions should include controls governing who is allowed inside the computer center, what signature approval is required to cause certain processing to take place, and what records must be made of computer center transactions.

Also, for the programming staff, instructions should state who is authorized to approve the commencement of an information systems project as well as who is authorized to make changes in software and under what conditions. Instructions should also state that no staff member is allowed to make personal use of the institution's data or software.

Employee training and competence

As with users of computer information systems, employees of the information services departments must be well informed and trained to limit exposure to mistakes. New computer systems are unfamiliar, and the general complexity of some computer concepts often causes employees to make errors. Here again, in light of the grave consequences of a serious mistake, this countermeasure is extremely important and merits high priority. As an extension of training, employees should periodically be tested for proficiency and retrained whenever necessary.

Management should particularly invest in improving information services employees' skills at choosing and planning controls for computer information systems. Information services professionals are typically assigned responsibility for selecting and designing controls for computer information systems, but these employees rarely develop appropriate high-level skills. As a result, they frequently design poor controls.

Controlling access to software libraries

Access to an institution's software library must be managed just as carefully as access to money in its bank accounts. These software libraries are the repositories from which a software program is invoked when required by scheduled computer processing, and a faulty software library could cause major errors in processing the institution's transactions. It is especially important to specify which employees have authority to access the software libraries to make changes, to enter new software into the libraries, and to copy or remove software from the libraries. Moreover, like bank accounts, computerized records of all transactions of software moved into and out of the libraries should be maintained to provide an audit trail that can be referenced if a problem or question subsequently arises.

One objective of controls on software libraries is to prevent mistakes that might be made by an uninformed person. Typically, the person seeking to make a change presents the proposed change to a manager. This manager either has authority to approve the change or must in turn seek the approval of a higher-level manager if the change's consequences are far-reaching enough to justify further review and approval.

Software library controls also seek to limit exposure to intentional corruption by an unauthorized person. Software library controls are the means, for example, to protect against the entry of software viruses that may be embedded in software from others' libraries. They are also a means to protect an institution from the unauthorized activities of a programmer who may otherwise have open access to the libraries and who could change a software program for personal financial benefit, carefully changing it back after the desired financial benefit has been realized.

An additional control objective centers on protecting software because it represents the intellectual property of the institution or of a vendor from whom the software is licensed. Effective software library controls prevent unauthorized people from making copies of software, printing the source code, and removing it from the premises for illegal use.

Preventing inappropriate access to data files

Like the software in software libraries, data in a health care institution's data files should be carefully managed. Protective data security barriers can be constructed to limit access to data files and to prevent accidental corruption of data, intentional unauthorized browsing, fraudulent modifications, and theft of data.

Special software packages are available that allow management to declare for each data file the staff members who are authorized to access the file and the conditions of access. For example, the master file of employee information can be controlled to allow access by certain specified staff members, by certain specified software programs, or by combinations of the two.

Supervision

Supervision of personnel in information services organizations is a very important preventive measure. The supervisor of a process in any one hospital department can no longer always exercise control over that entire process because the computer information system integrates the work of different hospital departments and masks the boundaries of people's work. Consequently, supervision of processes in the information services departments plays a vital role in providing the monitoring and assurance of quality that supervisors in other departments are unable to impose.

Strong supervision is the primary control over computer operations and computer programming personnel. Uncontrolled employees in these positions could potentially manipulate both computer software and data files to their own advantage, subsequently covering their tracks by restoring the software and files to their original form.

Physical location and physical security

Limiting physical access prevents unauthorized or incompetent personnel from causing computer information system problems. To control access, the primary computer processing equipment should be located in a computer center that has doors equipped with alarms and possibly with video camera surveillance. The computer center should be staffed at all times, and anyone who is not recognized as authorized should not be allowed to enter. Access should also be controlled to spaces such as wiring closets and office spaces containing computer system reference manuals and paper or microfiche copies of computer programs that must be quickly available for diagnosing and solving problems.

Scheduling and sequencing computer processing

Problems in computer production processing are usually caused by mistakes in judgment. Such problems can be limited by imposing effective controls over scheduling of computer processing.

One good control is to require that all computer processing be scheduled, specifically defining the detailed sequence and dependencies among processing steps. As much as 80 percent of processing can be preauthorized and scheduled far in advance.[12] Even when computer processing requirements arise on a shorter scheduling cycle, there is no reason why they cannot be formally scheduled before processing is authorized, both for consistency and to reap the benefits afforded by the review and careful preparation involved in scheduling. As a further reason to schedule all processing, formal analysis of any variances from the schedule provides reports that are useful in assessing exposure to problems caused by unscheduled processing.

Clearly separating the jobs of computer production scheduling and computer operations provides an additional effective control. The computer production scheduling and control group should be assigned the tasks of scheduling computer processing, thus ensuring that the data to be processed are available. After the scheduled computer processing is completed, this same group can review results to ensure that processing was correct, taking steps when necessary to remedy problems uncovered and following up to guarantee that incorrect or incomplete processing runs are rescheduled to resolve difficulties or errors.

Restart and reprocessing after an error is detected

When mistakes are made and computer processing errors uncovered, computer processing must usually be redone. Because error correction and reprocessing is often an error-prone activity, this process exposes the institution to a higher level of vulnerability. Reprocessing usually occurs under great time pressure and opens the institution to many vulnerabilities: software libraries are changed, data files are reset back to a state that existed prior to incorrect processing, and the computer processing is restarted at some previous intermediate processing point.

Consequently, this recovery activity and reprocessing of computer transactions must be subjected to more stringent controls than are applied to normal processing.[13] The recovery process must include management controls that limit confusion, that prevent decisions from being made by incompetent or unauthorized personnel, and that ensure maximum efficiency so that the system is functioning correctly again as soon as possible.

When a system fails and problems are uncovered, decisions are frequently made under pressure in the interest of getting processing on track quickly. Nightly patient accounting processing, for example, must be completed before patient accounting department employees can use the system the next day. Under the pressure of attempting to solve one problem, another problem could easily be caused, possibly only subtly affecting some data and therefore escaping detection for several days. To prevent such a chain reaction, controls must be introduced that limit the extent of activity authorized by each level of employee participating in problem-solving activity. For example, data security controls can prevent certain files from being restored to an earlier state unless authorized by a specific management level. Software library changes made during these special conditions must be reviewed immediately thereafter by management. Finally, automatic entry into a computerized log of all activities performed during this problem-solving period allows later reference if another problem arises, one that may have been caused by the original problem-solving activities.

Output distribution control guidelines

Distribution of computer output is another process that warrants close control. Timely and accurate delivery is important because many management processes depend on reports that must arrive promptly at correct locations. Additionally, confidential data must be handled sensitively during these activities.

Up-to-date distribution lists stating which reports are to be distributed to which people at which locations help to ensure accurate, timely distribution. This strategy's weakness, however, is that when people are relocated or reassigned, reports may still be distributed to old locations instead of, or in addition to, new locations. To avoid this problem, a report listing all employee reassignments and relocations can be produced and periodically compared against the list of report recipients, thereby allowing corrections to be made.

Additional control is provided by establishing a distribution schedule along with a job processing schedule, instead of simply distributing computer output as it becomes available. Such a control ensures that staff members know when reports should be distributed, and alerts them if a report is not available when expected. Requiring recipients to sign for receipt of certain material, especially if it is highly confidential, is another method of controlling output distribution.

Detective Countermeasures

Detective countermeasures minimize the extent of any damage that preventive countermeasures were unable to prevent. It is crucial that detective countermeasures be chosen and administered both to achieve early alerts when something is wrong and to provide quick diagnostic attention.

Environmental alarms

Environmental alarms provide early recognition of a causal agent's unusual presence, such as an unauthorized entry via an exit door or the existence of dangerous levels of smoke, dust, heat, static electricity, humidity, or water—any one of which could cause disastrous damage to the institution. Low humidity, for example, could cause static electricity to build up to a level that periodically affects the computer's electronic circuitry. Construction dust from nearby remodeling work could clog the air vents and moving parts of delicate disk storage equipment, causing it to fail. Poor air-conditioning circulation could mean that certain parts of the computer center receive less cooling than necessary, causing delicate heat-sensitive equipment to fail much more frequently than expected. Environmental alarms can also be used to detect unusual levels or changes in electrical power and chilled water supply to computer equipment.

Also, to maintain effectiveness, environmental alarms should be tested regularly. By the same token, training and testing of employees' knowledge of countermeasures should be conducted frequently and on all shifts. It is important that staff members fully understand the precise conditions that will activate alarms, as well as the precise steps required of them when an alarm does signal the presence of a causal agent.

Recording, analyzing, and tracking problems

Recording, analyzing, and tracking problems—an extension of the initial risk assessment process—focuses management's attention on the scope of problems encountered, especially those that continue or remain unresolved after a fairly long period. To determine potential impact on the institution, it is important that management analyze the kinds of computer system errors typically made and appraise the probable consequences.

To track and analyze these problems effectively, funnel all reports of problems to a central user assistance function (the help desk), where they can be recorded even if they are resolved immediately. All details of the problems should be recorded: date and time, system and system function involved, employee reporting the problem and his or her department, impact of the problem, to whom its correction is assigned, and action and progress notes leading to its resolution. A statistical summary of these recorded details can then be compiled and reviewed periodically to determine which problems occur most frequently and in which work areas. For example, traditional users of computer systems, such as registration departments, and newer users, such as nursing departments, often make different kinds of errors. Consequently, a long-term strategy for limiting problems may depend on both the types of problems occurring most frequently and the work areas in which they occur.

Reporting access to software libraries

As was mentioned in the discussion on preventive countermeasures, software libraries must be carefully controlled to limit (1) possibility of fraud, (2) potential corruption, either accidental or intentional, and (3) theft of intellectual property owned by the institution or by a software vendor. This particular vulnerability is so serious that, in addition to preventive countermeasures seeking to limit access, strong detective countermeasures must also be put in place. Specifically, record all accesses to provide an audit trail of programs that were copied from the libraries and of programs that were changed. The recorded data should include the time and date, the programs and version numbers affected, and the identification of the person who performed the access. Management can then easily review these details and determine whether it was logical for that person to make an authorized change to that program at that time of day and at that frequency. All new programs and purging of old programs should be scrutinized for possible vulnerability to fraudulent activities by members of the information services staff.

Reporting security password usage and nonusage

This is another case in which a strong detective countermeasure must supplement a strong preventive countermeasure. Because no preventive means of access control can completely prevent penetration, a compensating detective countermeasure should also be employed. The system should internally record all accesses, including the time and date, identification code, and terminal from which access occurred. Computerized reports should be periodically printed and reviewed, with a focus primarily on unusual patterns and unexpected combinations. For example, access to patient data from a computer terminal in the personnel department may be a combination worth examining.

Reports listing user identification codes that were not used recently help identify personnel that have been reassigned. After an appropriate time, unused access codes should be deactivated, requiring affected users to contact a control person and to arrange retraining before the codes are reactivated. After an additional period during which no request for reactivation is made, inactive user access codes should be purged.

Big Brother is watching: Special usage reports

As an extension of countermeasures detecting access to the system, it is also useful to provide a computer log that monitors and counts all occurrences of certain vulnerable transactions, recording the time and date, duration, user identification code, and terminal from which the transaction took place. For example, management may wish to detect how often certain exceptions take place, such as how often nursing orders are canceled by a treatment department. Or it may be helpful to monitor all transactions in a special class to determine how often they are used and to detect changes in usage patterns, such as how often physicians access certain functions to which they have access.

When this type of monitoring is used, management should inform users not only that a behind-the-scenes tracking mechanism is in place, but also why the processes are being monitored. Users who are so informed will not conclude that their privacy is being violated as the computer closely tracks what they are doing while they use the system.

Countermeasures that Lead to Corrective Action

A computer's automatic internal sensing and self-correction

Special features should be present within each system's software and hardware to internally detect improper processing, diagnose causes, and attempt correction, thereby sensing gradual degradation of the system and potentially permitting remedy before complete failure occurs. For example, computer systems can internally monitor the functioning of a degrading telephone line over which data are being transmitted to a remote building. The computer performs this monitoring by counting the frequency of errors that the system experiences over that line. As a corrective countermeasure, the system might automatically shift all transactions to an alternate telephone line while also alerting computer operations management to the existence of the degraded line.

Many computers have powerful self-correcting internal processes that detect failures, retry the internal process involved, and possibly complete the process successfully. These computers then automatically record the entire series of transactions (the error detected, the number of retries, and the eventual successful internal transaction) in a special internal file called a *log record* (sometimes abbreviated *logrec*). This data file should be analyzed frequently, both by computer center management and by vendor field maintenance representatives.

Automated fire alarm and suppression mechanisms

As a corrective countermeasure, the computer center and other locations housing critical computer equipment should be equipped with automatic fire detection and suppression mechanisms. Automated fire-inhibiting agents, such as Halon gas, can be used to inhibit combustion inside the computer center, while automated sprinkler systems in areas adjacent to the computer center can suppress fire and prevent its spread into the computer center. All automated fire alarms and fire suppression mechanisms must have engineered control mechanisms that allow for manual overrides so that they can be periodically tested or invoked manually if some automated component fails to operate properly.

Manual backup procedures

Another good corrective countermeasure involves designing procedures and forms that allow manual record keeping during any period when the computer cannot operate. For example, admitting department personnel might be instructed to record manually all patient room transfers on a form when the computer is unavailable, facilitating subsequent entry into the computer when it does become available. Or nursing personnel could record patient charges on a form so that they, too, can be entered later. An example of such a form was shown as Exhibit 7.2 in Chapter 7.

If such a process is used, however, additional controls must be defined to ensure accuracy at the two points of discontinuity: the shift from automated processing to manual processing, and the later shift from manual processing to automated processing. At these points of discontinuity, procedural flaws could allow some data transactions to be lost or entered twice. Use of prenumbered forms helps management account for each form used during the period of manual record keeping, ensuring, for example, that all charges are accounted for.

Redundant resources, backup, and disaster recovery

Redundancy of resources is an important countermeasure that is especially applicable to mechanical equipment that may require replacement parts from a distant site. For example, the inability to print computer output could be critical and, therefore, often justifies a backup printer. Similarly, a data communications unit that links nursing station computer terminals to the system may be critical enough to justify investment in a second unit, or a disk storage unit containing critical patient data may be sufficiently critical to justify redundant storage of critical data on two different disks. Also, sophisticated redundant electronic paths among computer equipment, such as between two computers in the same computer center or between computers and disk storage units, may be similarly justified.

At this level of sophistication, however, vulnerability shifts to the special mechanism that detects errors and invokes use of the redundancy. In the current state of the art, that special mechanism is usually singular, and its failure could cause unpredictable and catastrophic results. It can fail to sense errors that it should, for example, potentially corrupting processing or data without detection. It could also falsely detect errors that do not actually exist, or it could falsely sense that no valid paths or alternatives exist, incorrectly stopping processing when in fact there is no error in anything except the error detection mechanism.

To complement preventive and detective countermeasures, a recovery plan for major disruption of computer processing must be defined. Despite the protection provided by preventive and detective countermeasures, major failures of critical equipment, major damage, or disaster could still occur. The only remaining corrective countermeasure is to provide for recovery by processing on redundant computer equipment in another computer facility.

If some destructive event causes damage so devastating or outage so extensive that processing must be moved to an alternate site, the recovery plan must be invoked. The plan can specify an alternate site with computer facilities that will be immediately available and sufficient for processing. It should also specify which critical computer information system processing must be resumed first, as well as employees' responsibilities during this activity. The plan must be written and periodically tested, reevaluated, and revised so that it is not out of date. Responsible employees should also be thoroughly trained in their roles.

To support such a recovery plan, procedures must be formally established for periodically copying data files and software libraries and for storing those redundant copies off site. Procedures must also be established to ensure that paper copies of important reference material, such as printouts of the computer software source code, are available. The recovery plan should specify procedures for collecting these off-site data files, transporting them to the alternate site, and initiating processing there.

The comprehensive recovery plan should also specify procedures and responsibilities both for assessing damage to the primary facility, equipment, software, and files, and for beginning the necessary steps to repair and restore processing at the primary site.

Finally, it is also necessary to specify procedures for stopping or limiting use of the computer facility during local emergencies, such as loss of local electric power or water pressure, or during natural disasters, such as floods or hurricanes. Procedures should specify which equipment may be temporarily shut down and in what sequence, as well as minimum levels of service that will be provided during such a period.

Periodic audit

A periodic audit can be conducted of the computer processing facility and of information services staff functions, similar to that described earlier for the information systems themselves. Such a periodic audit not only helps determine whether controls over the computer processing and personnel procedures are defined and adhered to, but also helps assess their effectiveness.

Periodic audits provide an opportunity for management to reassess the vulnerabilities of the information services functions and the computer processing facility. At least one strong countermeasure should be in place for each major vulnerability; if not, several weaker complementing countermeasures could be equally effective.

Risk Management in Computer Information Systems

Management of computer information system risk is complex and formidable, but it is usually not included in job descriptions ascribed to institutional risk managers, who are responsible for monitoring and minimizing the institution's risk of substandard conformity to regulatory standards and subsequent penalties and malpractice claims. However, management of computer information system risk is as important as management of risk of institutional malpractice: an unrecoverable computer disaster could render the institution incapable of operating. To prevent such an occurrence, responsibilities must be assigned to an appropriate executive—and executive controls must be imposed to ensure that responsibilities are being accepted and fulfilled.

Assessing Risk

Before selecting appropriate countermeasures, management must first pinpoint critical areas where the institution is at the greatest risk and where effort is most justified. Risk assessment is performed to assess the threat of major causal agents: to determine the likelihood that such a causal agent will affect the institution, the consequences to the institution if that causal agent does have its effect at one or more points of vulnerability, the effort necessary to recover from those consequences, and the current countermeasure(s) present to limit vulnerability. Then, if necessary, an additional one or more counter-measures may be added to limit future vulnerability.

One simple way of beginning this process is to ask questions about the existence of protection against risks that would have great impact on the health care institution. The risks that one might think of very quickly would include risk of fraud or other financial loss, risk of patient care mistakes based on incorrect test results or other incorrect computerized data, and risk of noncompliance with data confidentiality principles and laws. Typical questions might include the following:

- What are the protections (countermeasures) against a dishonest em-ployee in either the information systems or accounting departments defrauding the hospital by receiving unauthorized accounts payable checks?

- What are the protections (countermeasures) against incorrect comput-erized patient test results being distributed for use, possibly leading to improper patient care?

- What are the protections (countermeasures) against someone obtain-ing copies of confidential patient data for unauthorized personal use, possibly for sale to others outside the hospital?

- What are the protections (countermeasures) against loss of use of the hospital's computer systems for an extended period of time?

- What are the protections (countermeasures) against unauthorized in-tentional access to computer systems by a hacker attempting trial-and-error access via telephone lines?

To assist in this process, the form shown in Exhibit 8.1 can be used to identify each causal agent and to list the hospital's vulnerability or, in many cases, the several vulnerabilities to this causal agent.[14] The form provides a convenient method for considering combinations of causal agents and vulner-abilities, and for describing countermeasures in place and those that might be added or substituted.

For the first example in the list above, in the "system and function" section of the form, the accounts payable system would be identified. Then, in the next section the causal agent (the dishonest employee) and the threat (defrauding the hospital by obtaining unauthorized accounts payable pay-ments) would be identified. In the next section, the several vulnerabilities would be listed, using one or more of the nine vulnerability numbers listed earlier in this chapter. One vulnerability is the possibility of the dishonest employee fraudulently causing a check to be addressed to some address that

Exhibit 8.1   Risk Assessment Form

Assessment of Causal Agents, Vulnerabilities, and Countermeasures

System and function:

Describe the threat and its causal agent:

Vulnerability number and description, countermeasures in place and
proposed additional countermeasures, type (preventive, detective, or
corrective), assessment of strength of each:

the employee has access to. An information systems employee could enter
the fraudulent invoice at many of the points of vulnerability described earlier.
To evaluate the risks, simply analyze each of the nine points of vulnerability.
For example, the employee could enter a fraudulent invoice at vulnerability
1 (unauthorized entry of the paper invoice into the work flow of accounting
people during data collection), or 2 (similar unauthorized entry during manual data movement), or 3 (unauthorized entry into the computer), or 4
(fraudulently changing data files inside the computer), or 5 (fraudulently
changing software to print a check for which no data entry was made). An
accounting employee could enter the fraudulent invoice only at vulnerabilities 1, 2, or 3, but not points 4 or 5, unless of course the employee had
computer programming skills and there were no countermeasures to prevent

an accounting person from gaining direct internal access to computer files and computer software libraries.

In the first example, there are other vulnerabilities, such as the possibility of someone simply stealing a check addressed to someone else, with the intention of forging it. In this case, the points of vulnerability include 6 (theft of a check during printing of checks), 7 (theft of a check during check distribution), and 8 (theft of a check from the user's work area).

Following the analysis of vulnerabilities, for each vulnerability exposed to the causal agent at least one countermeasure should be defined to limit the future risk.

The second example, involving incorrect patient test results, can be analyzed in the same way. In this case, as in the first, the causal agents include departmental staff, possibly poorly trained and accidentally making a mistake, or disgruntled and subverting a process. But the causal agent could also be an improperly functioning software program. The vulnerabilities should be analyzed in the same way as they were in the first example.

In the third example, involving someone obtaining confidential patient data for personal gain, the causal agent is again a person, and the vulnerabilities can be analyzed as they were in the first example.

In the fourth example, involving loss of use of the computer system itself, the causal agent could be people; computer hardware or software malfunction; loss of a utility, such as electricity or telecommunications access; or a disaster due to a hurricane, tornado, fire, or flood. Here again, the vulnerabilities should be analyzed for each causal agent that involves people. But, for the types of causal agents that do not involve people, the only vulnerability that applies is vulnerability 5, loss of computer processing itself. To address the variety of potential causal agents that might result in total loss of use of the computer system, a good place to start is to ask questions regarding all the computer system problems that occurred during the past month.

In the fifth example, the threat is unauthorized access from outside over telephone lines, and the causal agent is a person. The several vulnerabilities, such as vulnerability 3, entry of unauthorized data into the system, can be analyzed as they were in the first example. Exhibit 8.2 shows a completed Risk Assessment Form for the fifth example, assessing the risk of intentional unauthorized access by a hacker outside the institution.

It is not practical to complete such a form for every combination of causal agent and vulnerability, but it is important to assess risk for those combinations that appear most likely to occur and that would result in the greatest loss to the health care institution. Other combinations can later be considered when their importance becomes apparent.

Exhibit 8.2 Completed Risk Assessment Form

Assessment of Causal Agents, Vulnerabilities, and Countermeasures

System and function:

Hospital information system and all systems allowing dial-in access from outside hospital.

Describe the threat and its causal agent:

Unauthorized intentional access by a hacker on the outside with a personal computer and modem with which he or she may attempt to use a trial-and-error process to gain access to functions, possibly obtain confidential data, and possibly corrupt data in the system.

Vulnerability number and description, countermeasures in place and proposed additional countermeasures, type (preventive, detective, or corrective), assessment of strength of each:

- **Vulnerability 3. Entry of unauthorized data into the computer system.**

  - **Countermeasures in place:** Call-back unit to prevent access from a phone number not previously defined in the system and associated with a specific user code (a very strong preventive control). However, if a hacker were able to achieve access to an authorized computer terminal, possibly to the office of an authorized user in the off-hours, a preventive control would limit access to three trial-and-error attempts to use unauthorized combinations of codes and passwords before requiring redialing. Detective controls would detect a large number of redials, alerting management to the location and time of the unauthorized physical access to an office. If the hacker using an authorized terminal were to know and use an authorized code and password, preventive controls would limit access to the functions and data normally available to the authorized user. Detective controls would detect the period of access and, if it were lengthy, raise questions about the appropriateness of the time and duration.

  - **Proposed additional countermeasures:** Special reports of all access from off-site locations after 6 p.m. longer than 10 minutes, routed to the management of the office area for review.

- **Vulnerability 6. Confidential data being exposed to unauthorized person.**

  - **Countermeasures in place:** Same as above.

  - **Proposed additional countermeasures:** Same as above.

- **Vulnerability 3. Entry of software virus into software library.**

  - **Countermeasures in place:** Access controls same as above. Additional controls prevent entry of additions to software libraries by anyone except those with special management-level passwords.

Continued

Exhibit 8.3 Continued

- **Proposed additional countermeasures:** If an unauthorized person were to penetrate all access controls and in addition gain access to a management-level password, access would be possible. An added control would be to require that verbal agreement be obtained with the computer operations supervisor, who would converse with the person on the telephone and verify their identity and authorization.

- **Vulnerability 6. Piracy of owned or vendor software.**

- **Countermeasures in place:** Same as above.

- **Proposed additional countermeasures:** Same as above.

Balancing Countermeasures for Appropriate Protection

Once a major risk is identified, management must impose suitable counter-measures that limit vulnerabilities and guarantee continued functioning of the institution's computer systems. For example, if a hospital were to lose access to its computer systems, or if the accuracy and credibility of its data were to be eroded, the institution would not have access to information necessary to administer care to its patients. On the other hand, unreasonable barriers must not be imposed. Relatively easy access should be available to all who have need and authority. Countermeasures should therefore be balanced and adapted to the magnitude of each threat.

Notes

1. B. Minard, "Full-Time, Real-Time System Security," *Computers in Healthcare* (October 1987): 51–57.
2. W. Mair et al., *Computer Control and Audit* (Altamonte Springs, FL: The Institute of Internal Auditors, 1978), pp. 12–13.
3. R. Fisher, *Information Systems Security* (Englewood Cliffs, NJ: Prentice-Hall, 1984), pp. 51–62.
4. Ibid., p. 55.
5. Ibid., pp. 57–62.
6. Mair, *Computer Control and Audit,* pp. 69–75.
7. Ibid., p. 86.
8. Minard, "Full-Time, Real-Time System Security," pp. 55–57.
9. B. Minard, "Modern Principles Improve Information Systems," *Healthcare Financial Management* (June 1988): 140–44.

10. Minard, "Full-Time, Real-Time System Security."
11. Fisher, *Information Systems Security,* pp. 104–5
12. Mair, *Computer Control and Audit,* pp. 324–25.
13. Ibid., p. 88.
14. Fisher, *Information Systems Security,* pp. 138–41.

9

THE INFORMATION ADVANTAGE: MANAGING DATA AS AN IMPORTANT RESOURCE

In much the same way that a library is concerned with collecting, storing, planning, managing, and providing access to books and other reference materials, information resources management is concerned with collecting, storing, planning, managing, and providing access to information entrusted to a computer information system. Moreover, just as libraries rely on systematic, orderly procedures to manage their collections effectively, so health care institutions require sound procedures governing the organized collection and assimilation of data from which critical information will be gleaned.

A New Era: The Information-Based Organization

Computer speed and capacity have made it possible to collect and store great amounts of data beyond the health care institution's immediate needs. This storage capability, in turn, has prompted clinicians and management to expect computers to assimilate data and make them available for later reference, as opposed to merely storing data that are incidental to immediate processing requirements. As a result, health care institutions will increasingly collect more data, save them longer, and give more people access to them.

The challenge of managing information during this new era is to collect and store the right data, ensure data quality, provide the capability to exchange data among computer information systems, organize the stored data for use in comprehensive analyses, and channel relevant information to appropriate management and clinical personnel on a timely basis.

The dramatically changing health care business environment has sparked new emphasis on case management, product line management, diversification toward outpatient and aftercare services, clinical information systems at the point of care, and market competition in cost and quality. Health care institutions that are to thrive in this dynamic environment must plan to collect new data and integrate them with existing data in order to provide a data repository from which comprehensive management and clinical analyses can be obtained.

Data must be managed as an important resource. They are fast becoming the basis for important health care decisions and the foundation for the decision support systems and executive information systems that will soon be sought by all institutions.

Including a Wide Scope of Data

Data are so available that the very availability has become an issue. Most health care information systems have evolved without broad planning for the use of data integrated from several operational computer systems. Consequently, large amounts of data that are redundantly collected and stored, and duplicated in several overlapping data cycles and computer systems, are the basis for paper reports distributed widely throughout the health care institution. Occasional ambiguities in some data subtly discredit the value of all data. Moreover, people have become inundated with paper and suffer from information overload.

Health care management and clinicians must therefore accept the challenge of deciding which data are to be stored in the institution's computerized data bases and for what they will be used. The initial step in this process, determining what data are needed, must anticipate future as well as current needs.

Information that Answers Traditional Management Questions

Effective monitoring of a health care institution's operations usually depends on the availability of standard monthly reports comparing performance with a budget or plan. However, these traditional monthly financial and management reports leave many relevant questions unanswered.

Data in the data base should provide an effective means for analyzing issues of traditional management concern. If salaries are over budget, for example, the data base should include data necessary to identify departments with the greatest budget variance and also to analyze their trends over a period of time. If supply costs are over budget, a similar analysis of departmental supply costs should be possible—and the data base should allow analysis of trends over a period of time.

The data base should also include data that facilitates analysis of traditional management questions relating to employees, salaries, and productivity. For example, if a department suffers from high levels of overtime, excessive turnover, or other productivity or personnel problems, data should be available for analyses of recent salary transactions, the position of individual salaries within salary ranges, performance appraisal trends, trends of departmental hours worked by shift, departmental procedures performed by shift, and other potentially relevant trends.

Data necessary to analyze the departmental work of clinical departments should also be included in the data base. If management is concerned about departmental revenue fluctuations or interdepartmental work flow difficulties that appear to be influencing services to patients, management will need access to data such as average time between placement of orders and service, number of orders canceled, number of orders left unfilled at the ends of shifts, and recent trends for each of these and similar work items.

Answering a New Category of Questions: Computerized Data in Support of the Clinical Diagnostic Process

Computerized medical records are slowly becoming a reality. Paper records will still be used, but computers are recording an increasing amount of important clinical data: orders, results, patient transfers among rooms and nursing units, patient charges, materials and medications used, diagnoses at various stages of care, tests and procedures performed, DRGs assigned, severity of illness, intensity of nursing care, duration and other facts about surgical cases, and other details concerning inpatient or outpatient encounters. These recorded data serve as a computerized subset of the medical record and can become part of the computerized data base from which important new analytical information is obtained.

A data base integrating these data from the several computer systems of the health care institution can support patient care directly. It can provide clinicians easy-to-use, timely, and relevant computer-assisted analysis of data as they diagnose and treat their patients.

Such a data base can also provide access for clinical research purposes, provided that proper data confidentiality controls are applied to preserve patients' rights of privacy. In the case of research access, the question of data ownership arises, since clinicians traditionally may have believed that data in separate clinical or departmental data bases have been available for research, free of institutional controls. New institutionwide data controls must be defined, negotiated, and accepted, in an ongoing process.[1]

Answering a New Category of Questions: Cost and Quality of Outcomes of Medical Cases

Health care's new analytical information needs demand information that analyzes cost and its interdependency with quality of care.[2] Cost analysis relies on information regarding costs for procedures, comparisons with standards, costs by case, and costs correlated with the quality of outcomes of cases. Such determinations are vital for basic management analyses; these same cost and quality analyses are also useful to present to employers and payers to attract buyers and consumers of care. Yet another reason for gathering this information is to perform analyses to pinpoint the extent to which revenue, cost, and profitability are influenced by internal and external factors. Internal factors include the institution's policies and procedures, productivity, management, and medical practices. External factors are those characteristic of the patient population, such as demographics, severity of illness, and cost of materials and services.

New health care information requirements additionally encompass indepth analysis of patient cases for quality assurance purposes. Comprehensive analysis of data on patient cases provides information that in turn could prompt alerts of clinical significance, such as identifying cases of one particular physician that deviate significantly from those of peers in cost per case, length of stay, or other pertinent measure. Comprehensive analysis of patient cases can also yield important facts about product line trends, along with other market analysis information.

Analysis of outcomes of medical cases, for either cost or quality analysis, will likely trigger some negative reactions by physicians, who may conclude that the computerized data will be used to monitor their practice of medicine. On this issue, as on others, communication with the physicians is important, to assure the physicians that the data will not be passed to others, and that use of the data for detailed analyses, such as for statistical or other research analyses, will be properly controlled. They must be assured that access to the data will be prevented unless authorized, and that authorized users' access will be responsibly monitored.

Defining and Managing the Data Base Contents

Health care institutions have experienced many difficulties while seeking to define the scope of data to be stored and managed. Some have collected too much of the wrong data; others have collected too little of the right data. It can be extremely difficult to define which data are necessary: data requirements change rapidly and depend on personal decision styles, which frequently change as managers and clinical personnel grow in their jobs or change positions.[3]

Data requirements for some hospital functions are more easily defined because these functions are traditional and relatively stable, such as financial management. Moreover, research has shown that the lower the level of management, the easier the task of defining data requirements.[4] However, data requirement decisions are much more difficult when the targeted clinical or management function encompasses complex interdependencies. Long-range hospital planning, for example, requires data from many different departments.[5]

Data base content is usually administered by a project team or other group responsible for information resources management (IRM). The IRM staff also performs other tasks: managing the technical structure and physical storage of the files, managing data security and access to data, and providing instruction and assistance in use of data in the data base. IRM staff members must possess a detailed understanding of the tasks, users, and management processes that the data base supports. Assigned IRM staff members identify organizational information needs and define data elements to be included in the data base, including the operational process from which each data element is to be derived (for example, patient registration), the data cycle in which the data element is collected (for example, monthly), and the department that generates the data element (for example, the patient registration department). In theory, the task should also include definition of the processes in which each data element is used (for example, DRG reimbursement and various reports). However, it is generally not practical to document all potential uses of data elements because such usage is inherently so dynamic and likely to change frequently.

To pinpoint which data should be included in the data base, the importance of each type of data must be determined. This can be accomplished by defining the data required for important functions, such as using of patient test results in patient care, evaluating market share, analyzing pricing trends, or evaluating performance of executives. An alternate method involves listing the health care institution's critical success factors,[6] defined by the CEO and other senior executives, and selecting key numerical indicators based on those factors. Necessary data elements can then be defined, from which key indicators can be calculated and critical success factors can be monitored.

Finally, because data content must continuously evolve, the IRM staff will continue to define both changes necessary in data base content and procedures for collecting new or changed data. One key to the IRM staff's success lies in its ability to extend the data base quickly and easily, adapting it to new uses and new users.

Internal Sources of Data

Internal operations are the principal source of data for the data base. Financial (and administrative) systems provide data such as patient registration data, patient orders, patient charges, patient transfers, departmental statistics, medical record abstracting data, operating room statistics, patient acuity data, and any other administrative and financial data recorded about inpatient or outpatient encounters. Data from clinical systems include medications ordered and administered, the results of patient tests, and data from nursing information systems. As more and more clinical processes are automated to produce computer records of test results, the data base will contain more and more of patients' medical records. In consolidating these data, data cycles must be coordinated so that data are collected once and once only, avoiding possible ambiguity that is created when data are recorded twice or are missed altogether.

Data will ultimately take forms other than the standard uppercase characters typical in today's computer reports. Lowercase characters are now being used more often, and images and even digitized voice records will eventually be suitable for storage in data bases.

External Sources of Data

Many companies, such as Dun & Bradstreet, Dow Jones, McGraw-Hill, and Mead Corporation, are creating what is coming to be known as the information industry. They electronically gather information from many sources—health care insurance claims, personal credit records, stock markets, and other markets—and then electronically distribute that information to customers who find it valuable. These firms are essentially information brokers: information in their commercial data bases is a commodity for sale.

With such information, a health care institution can analyze estimates of per capita incomes and spending, health care insurance claims trends, and local demographics trends such as population growth rates and residents' ages and family sizes.

Customers of these information industry firms can subscribe to selected information services. The data may be mailed to customers regularly on a magnetic tape or diskette, or customers may gain access to data by connecting a personal computer in their own offices through a dial-up telephone line connection to a computer on which the commercial data bases reside. Costs are usually based on usage, such as the duration of time that the personal computer is connected to the service. Collected data can be temporarily stored on the personal computer and then consolidated and integrated with data collected from other sources.

Quality and Credibility

A decision is only as good as the information on which it is based. The problem today is not lack of information, it is lack of information quality. Data bases often include data that are inaccurate, ambiguous, outdated, untimely, or irrelevant. Users consequently suffer from the inability to distinguish between data that are useful and data that are not.

Measures of Data Quality

Several dimensions of data quality exist, but research has shown that users usually cannot or do not differentiate among these dimensions. For example, data quality depends on accuracy, relevance, clarity of definition and how well the data content is understood, timeliness, consistency and synchronization among sources, and accessibility.[7] Users tend to draw conclusions about quality and value without distinguishing among the several measures of quality.

The same research has established that, in general, relevance and timeliness are more important than accuracy. However, at lowest levels of management, accuracy seems to be the most important data characteristic. At intermediate levels, concern is directed at timeliness and consistency; at executive levels, concern centers on drawing relevant and proper interpretations from the data.

Data Edits for Accuracy

Data edits include special computerized controls that guarantee data's accuracy and completeness. Edits are applied by computer software as data are entered into a computer information system, and they ensure quality by verifying the validity of details (such as dates, charge codes, and permutations of charge codes and cost centers) and by confirming that numerical values (such as patient test results) are within reasonable limits.

Special edits are usually also applied if more than one department or organizational group makes active, simultaneous use of the same data elements. To prevent integrity problems that can arise when users make unilateral changes unknown to other users and potentially affecting their work, specific controls are imposed to govern the updating of each data element in the data base. These controls allow and disallow updating by certain users and during certain periods, thus preserving data integrity, accuracy, and consistency. For example, a clinical lab computer system may receive patient demographic data automatically from another computer, but special software within that clinical lab computer includes special edits that control the updating of those patient demographic data once they become resident within the lab computer system. Because the patient demographic data may not be updated independently of the main computer, the patient demographic data are the same in the two computers. Similarly, clinical data transferred from a clinical system to a data base in another computer system are not allowed to be updated independently of the clinical system from which they came.

Consistent and Clear Definition of Data Elements

To safeguard data quality, controls can also be imposed to ensure that data elements are clearly defined and well understood. This approach, especially important among distributed computer systems, prevents data from becoming misinformation through misunderstandings about data contents or inappropriate interpretations of data analyses.

Defining each data element in a published data dictionary creates a permanent base for consistent usage throughout the health care institution. By eliminating ambiguity of meaning, the data dictionary ensures that each data element has the same meaning to all personnel who make use of it. The data dictionary additionally provides an invaluable catalog of all available data.

Dictionaries can also be used to include definitions of standard codes employed in the data base, such as those for identifying nursing stations, discharge dispositions, and local employers. These codes eliminate potential ambiguity of text data. When the local First National Bank, for example, is entered into a computer system as a patient's employer under its entire name, or abbreviated as First National, or perhaps even FNB, the likelihood exists that the same employer may appear to be several different employers, eroding the accuracy of reports of patients' employers. If, on the other hand, a unique code is assigned to the bank, the risk of entering the bank in different ways so that it appears to be several different employers is eliminated.

Data elements that are standardized have a consistent meaning over time, and they mean the same to the person retrieving data as to the person collecting and entering data. For example, individual department managers should be required to conform to institutional guidelines for defining and reporting departmental work units; they should not be free to change the meanings of work units, such as procedures performed, for example. Without such enforced standardization, a "procedure" might be arbitrarily defined differently by different department managers. Ambiguously defined, a lab test in one department might be counted as one procedure while in another it might be considered to be ten separate procedures, even though it is managed as one unit of manual work (one order or one specimen).

Problems stemming from data aggregation from several data bases in distributed computers are fast becoming one of the biggest roadblocks to effective corporate use of data bases.[8] In order to help solve these problems, data definitions should be consistent across data in distributed computer systems, if possible. For example, a data element such as patient name in a pathology computer system should have the same format and characteristics as the data element for patient name in the main hospital information system and other clinical systems, such as a radiology or pharmacy computer system. In addition, data dictionaries should identify differences among similar data elements or data elements derived from one another, such as data collected from one computer system and summarized and transferred to be stored in another computer system. Consistency of data elements across distributed computers is a major issue that must be addressed if data bases, decision support systems, and executive information systems are to be effective.

Similarly, data elements should also be standardized across the systems of several vendors. Unfortunately, even though most vendors of computer information systems used in health care institutions specialize in health care computer systems, such data element characteristics seldom match.

Finally, although consistency among data elements is a necessary goal, it can never be fully achieved in practice. Temporary inconsistencies will arise and must therefore be acknowledged and managed, with both the dictionary and the data base in a continuous state of change.

Data Cycles and Data Transfer

As information is aggregated by transferring data from several distributed computer systems to others on different time cycles, errors can be introduced easily. For example, data may be stored redundantly as they are transferred from more than one source, such as from medical records abstracting and patient registration data sources. Or the unsynchronized timing of data transfers may result in incomplete data in the data base, such as occurs when patient charges are included for some departments but are absent or late arriving for others.

Transfer of data to the data base should consequently be controlled and synchronized to ensure both that data are transferred correctly and that all required data are transferred. Various data transfer options are available. Data can be transferred whenever they are updated, such as whenever a new patient is registered. Or they can be transferred only when requested, such as whenever a specific test result is retrieved by a physician's office. Finally, data can be transferred only on a preset schedule, such as transferring batches of agreed-upon data at the end of each day. In any case, there must be some method for specifically authorizing all data transfers. The authorization may be imbedded as a specification in the computer information system's design. Or the data transfer may be specifically scheduled. Or it may be invoked through a special software feature that allows a window of access for data transfer, requires special approval for retransfer, and alerts management when data are not transferred on schedule.

Data Management

Data can be synthesized into valuable information only when considerable effort is invested in organizing the data and making them available to people who will use them. A data base of consolidated data must therefore be carefully organized and managed. This need may justify the acquisition and use of a formal software package known as a data base management system (DBMS) that organizes and manages large quantities of complex data. Such software is expensive and requires skilled staff for effective use, however. As in other management activities, work organized for the convenience of others demands investment of resources.

Basic Data Management Functions

The objective of data base management is to keep track of stored data, including the dictionary-like name by which the data are to be referenced, the physical location, and other characteristics. Computer software is required to perform these tasks, which include processing the data transferred to the data base, determining where to store the data, controlling access to reading and writing of data, and archiving or otherwise disposing of data that are displaced or otherwise beyond usefulness.

Technical Structure

The term *data base* is used both to refer conceptually to the organized and stored data (as it has been used thus far in this chapter) and to refer collectively to physically stored data files that are organized to contain the data. A physical data base includes many *data elements,* each of which contains one piece of information, such as a patient's name. Groups of related data elements are stored together as one *record,* such as the patient's name, birth date, and other demographic data. Groups of related records are stored together as a *file,* such as patient registration data on all patients. Several files in combination form a physical *data base,* and special cross-referenced indexes define *relationships* among the data elements, records, and files, making possible organized retrieval of information.

A data base is usually organized as one large, centrally located repository for all data, although an alternative concept of a large data base distributed over several computer systems is emerging in the marketplace. DBMSs provide technical structure for the internal organization and handling of data within a data base. The technical structure in turn determines both efficiency of processing and ease of retrieving data from the data base.

The principal difference among vendors' DBMS products lies in the method of maintaining indexing and cross-referencing relationships among data elements in the data base. For example, the technical structure of some DBMS products requires little computer processing effort to organize data as they are loaded. These systems simply organize data in its natural *hierarchical* form, such as organizing all charges with an episode of illness and organizing these episodes with patient identification data. However, these software products require significant computing resources to selectively retrieve data as a member of a set (such as all patients with the same diagnosis). Other DBMS products invest computing resources in storing the data together with its *relational* characteristics (so as to be able to retrieve all patients with the same diagnosis), resulting in easier and more rapid retrieval.

Both types of data base software products have advantages. Hierarchical data bases are commonly used to support traditional processing of the hospital's financial, administrative, and clinical transactions, and they support them well. On the other hand, relational data bases more effectively serve decision-support processes that must analyze varied subsets of data elements. Some health care institutions use both types: a hierarchical data base for support of normal daily processing and a relational data base into which data are copied for complex data analyses.

Either type of DBMS software package requires significant support personnel and other resources. Considerable learning and skill are necessary both to define data structures and to manage the data loading and data transfer processes. Additionally, appropriate amounts of computerized data storage space must be made available, and they must be adequate for the continuous growth that results as more and more data are added to the data base. Data files must also be carefully managed within the data base so that heavily used files are readily available internally, just as an office worker would store ready-reference material in a desk drawer while less-used material might be stored more remotely in a nearby filing cabinet. Because of the high levels of skill and management involved, use of DBMS software packages has evolved very slowly from their inception in the 1960s. Moreover, they have not been as useful as was first expected.

Data bases are usually stored on electromagnetic disk storage units. New generations of electromagnetic disk storage units allow data to be more densely stored, placing more and more data characters in increasingly smaller physical spaces. A new optical disk storage technology is now emerging, however, that allows data to be stored even more densely, dramatically extending the amounts of data that can be stored and referenced.

Data Relationships and Structure

Prestructuring data

Effectiveness in amassing data and making them useful depends to some extent on how well a pattern of retrieval requests is anticipated when the data base is designed. In efforts to organize data so that they are most accessible and flexible, data base designers must choose between storing data at the simplest level or partially prestructuring data to appear in the form and level of detail that will be required by anticipated requests.[9]

Several prestructuring alternatives exist. Data can be prestructured for case analysis, anticipating detailed breakdown of patient data by DRG, ICD-9, or other disease category. The same data can be structured for use by physicians—prestructured, for example, by physician, patient, procedures performed, and date and time. The same data can also be prestructured for cost accounting to perform analysis of patient data by hospital department, building, job code, or work shift. Or the data can be prestructured for product line analysis, which is oriented toward analyzing revenue, costs, and margin in each product line. Alternatively, data can be prestructured to permit examination of quality of patient care outcomes, tapping the data base for measures of illness severity and anticipating analysis by service, physician, and possibly nursing unit.

The challenge here lies in defining a data organization that maximizes the data repository's usefulness to those who will retrieve and analyze data. Each data element could, consequently, be defined to be retrievable by several identifiers: patient (that is, the ability to retrieve all information about a given patient), physician (that is, retrieve information about all the cases of any given physician), subsidiary corporation of the health care institution (if the institution is a multihospital system), payer, local employer, DRG, disease category, nursing stations where patient care was delivered, medical service, historical time period, geographic region, and referral source. Depending on anticipated usage, other identifying characteristics might also be appropriate.

Ownership and responsibility

The data in the data base are derived from the health care institution's operational transactions, and claims of departmental ownership and implicit control of the data may arise. Data ownership is often claimed by the department performing the work that creates the data, such as a clinical department that generates patient test results or a financial department that is responsible for monthly processing on which financial reports are based. However, the health care institution itself should be declared the sole owner of data—not individual departments—and data should not be withheld from reasonable access by others in the institution. Formal procedures can be implemented to allow appropriate data access from across departmental boundaries. For example, accountability for data accuracy should remain with the department that created the data. And, when multiple departments make use of the data, only one department should have the authority to correct or otherwise change data, and then only under strict controls. Such policies ensure that others are aware of any changes and also understand their purpose and significance.

Distributed data bases

As computer interconnections proliferate, and as computer processing on mainframe computers, minicomputers, and personal computers blends together, data are often collected on one computer but must be made available to other computers. Data may be physically stored on one computer and retrieved from another, or physical copies of data may be transferred to other computers. Between these two extremes lie various other methods of sharing data among computers.

Many health care institutions currently rely on methods of sharing data that were principally determined by the vendors selected for departmental clinical computer systems. For example, in many cases minicomputers were selected for radiology department computer systems because they could be implemented easier and more quickly than mainframe systems. More recently, however, personal computer solutions are being selected because they allow the technology to be implemented easier and more quickly than minicomputer systems. Each installed system has capabilities and limitations that determine how data will be shared or transferred.

Researchers have determined that vendors' technology should no longer be the primary criterion for deciding how data should be consolidated or decentralized; instead, the health care institution's management methods and critical needs should be considered.[10] For example, a large central data base should be selected when the data base is so large that only mainframe-based disk storage units are practical. A large central data base also allows greater centralized control, if that is necessary or desired. On the other hand, a distributed single copy of a data base can provide for simpler control by the department responsible for data accuracy. A large central data base provides easier access by an extensive group of users, in addition to better control of standards and integrity. Nevertheless, a distributed data base may be a wiser choice where data access is not likely to be required outside one department.

When a data base does exist in distributed form, controls can be imposed to prevent corruption of data integrity. First, a consolidated view of the entire partitioned data base should be made available through dictionaries. Additionally, if data are copied and stored in other data bases, one of the two or more versions of the data should be declared as the master while the others are designated as the copies. Rigid procedures must be established to ensure that any change made to the master is also made to the copies. Then, if differences appear between the two or more versions, the master data base can be used to resolve any ambiguity.

But even with such management principles in place, data integrity problems inevitably occur. Modern spreadsheet software for use in personal computers encourages users to obtain private versions of data for analysis. Data could be copied from another computer on a computer network, for example, or downloaded from large data bases in larger computers. Such uncontrolled movement of data often creates problems. Data could be copied incorrectly, or copied data could be superseded by later changes. Compounding the problem, subsequent copies of already copied data could be distributed to others. Technology is capable of providing some solutions to these problems, but by far the most practical solution now available is for management both to provide sound procedures and controls that specify which subsets of data can be replicated and to establish methods of communications that alert potential users when the master copy of replicated data is changed.

Usage: The Right Data to the Right Person at the Right Time

In the face of information overload, the bottom-line objective must be to simplify access to data so that they can be used to produce valuable information that benefits the health care institution. In the final analysis, the data available are not as important as the use that is made of them: providing timely and accurate information to management and to clinicians. In other words, the right data must be made available to the right person at the right time.

Decision Support Systems for Clinicians, Managers, and Executives

Decision support systems for managers or clinicians

Decisions are made by acting on information. High-quality information reduces uncertainty so that better decisions can ultimately be made. The term *decision support system* (DSS) was coined to describe a type of system providing information that supports managers' or clinicians' decisions.[11] These end-user systems typically allow easy on-line retrieval and analysis of data. The analysis usually leads to additional questions, which then can be answered by continued access to the same data base. In this circular process, access to data creates questions and ideas, which allow the decision maker to think about the results, create a new set of questions, and receive a new set of answers, ultimately leading to decisions.

For management decision making, case management data bases are good examples of such data bases. Data collected from a range of operational and clinical systems allow management analysis, for example, of reimbursement trends by payer, cost, product line profitability, productivity of departments, and reimbursement by referral source.

For clinical decision making, the computerized medical record data, and possibly even the case management data bases, will be useful. Aggregated patient data, such as data about patient tests, results, medications, diagnoses, and sensitivities, may be correlated and examined for information that would be useful to clinicians for planning patient care.

Executive support systems

A variation of a decision support system, called an *executive information system* (EIS) or an *executive support system,* is emerging and is expected to be used directly by senior executives, possibly by the CEO.[12] Such systems are based on the same types of data as are decision support systems and provide executives with the kind of information they previously—and frequently—had to procure from someone else. An EIS generally includes large numbers of key indicators and, to be successful, must be very easy to use.

Executive information systems usually provide two functions: access to key indicators of business performance and the capability to analyze beyond those key indicators. The challenge of implementing an effective EIS lies in the painstaking process of carefully defining key indicators along with the data elements and algorithms that will produce those key indicators.

An EIS changes the way that information flows to executive levels of management, potentially breeding some hostility in the ranks of middle management. EIS information no longer percolates its way up a long hierarchical chain and, consequently, is not merged with decisions made along the way. Use of an EIS causes the data on which decisions are based to be scrutinized at higher levels, where an executive might ask additional analytical questions to verify that all implications are understood and evaluated and may be more likely to question decisions made by others. Middle-level managers may act differently when they know that the numbers are being examined closely at the top, having bypassed their potential screening.

As the system presents key indicator data, executives must be able to analyze the data behind any indicator. Such a capability is sometimes called a *drill down capability*. When the system highlights an indicator out of normal range, or the executive considers some indicator trending in a new direction, the system allows the executive to drill down to lower levels of data on which that indicator depends until the desired degree of detail is reached.

Critics of executive information systems argue that the value of these systems is severely limited. They assert that most top-level executives do not and will not accept the notion that their job involves searching through key indicators to locate problems and gain information through the system to initiate action that will lead to problem resolution. The critics contend that such searching and analysis is a staff job, as is the job of drilling down and reanalyzing until the problem and its solution emerge.

The Right Data in the Right Amount

Appropriate data for managers and executives could include a variety of performance indicators: revenue, deductions from revenue, fixed and variable costs, indicators of employee and departmental productivity, hospital utilization, and quality of outcomes of patient care. Similar indicators, such

cians. The data might also, for each indicator, include variability of outliers on both sides of the norm, and developing trends.

But how can any institution determine exactly which information should be provided to its managers, executives, and clinicians? Various answers to this question have been proposed throughout the history of use of information systems by managers and executives, and all generally involve either asking the managers, executives, and clinicians, or telling them.[13,14] In one approach, these potential users are interviewed and asked what information they want, which is then provided. Another approach involves conducting a study of managers', executives', and clinicians' work processes and decision processes; they are then provided information necessary to support those processes. In another approach, called the by-product approach, these potential users are simply sent whatever available information lower-level personnel choose to send. In the null approach, users are assumed to operate on oral reports and special one-time reports, so no systematic data are prepared. In the key indicator approach, certain key indicators of interest to the managers, executives, and clinicians are provided on a predetermined cycle. In the prototyping approach, samples of data are provided to determine which data really matter and who needs which data. In yet another approach, the critical success factor method, each potential user defines a limited number of critical factors on which the health care institution's successful competitive performance depends. From those critical factors, appropriate data indicators are determined.

In all these approaches, the great quantity of data provided is a common problem. Computer technology seems to have overwhelmed institutions not only with a great quantity of data and reports, but also with options and flexibility of data availability. As a result, information is only partially used—and much of what is used is not the most relevant.

One dimension of data quantity involves whether data should be available in detailed form or summarized form. Another dimension centers on whether data should cover the immediate short-term period or a longer period over which trends can be determined. Researchers scrutinizing these dimensions have concluded that information overload is a major problem and, consequently, that strategies providing smaller amounts of data are more effective. One study examined the effect that information quantity had on the speed of people's decisions and their confidence in those decisions. It found that a group using summarized data took longer to make decisions and was less confident; however, it made better decisions. On the other hand, the group using detailed data had more difficulty identifying a problem and also more difficulty in resolving that problem once it was identified.[15] Another study found that subjects already overwhelmed with information actually

study found that subjects already overwhelmed with information actually continued to request more information than was necessary.[16]

In a similar study focusing on the amount of data made available to decision makers, an independent variable was introduced to determine the effect, if any, of uncertainty in the working environment, such as might be the case in clinicians' use of data.[17] Dependent variables included the degree of aggregation in the data made available, confidence in the decisions made, the amount of additional information requested, and effectiveness of decisions made.

Results of this study indicated preferences for data among three distinct groups. The group that had very little uncertainty in their working environment preferred summary information for a short historical period, possibly because they were confident of their working environment and focused on the short term. In contrast, the group that had medium uncertainty in their working environment preferred the greatest quantity of information, choosing detailed information for a long historical period. Finally, the group with high levels of uncertainty in their working environment preferred detailed information for a short historical period, probably because they felt the situation was so dynamic that the long term did not matter and was not as accessible as the short term. This last group wanted detailed, short-term data to gain insight with which to formulate decisions.

Results of this study also indicated that frequency of requests for data was consistent among the three groups, that effectiveness of decisions was only weakly related to amount and frequency of information, and that confidence in results was weakly related to amount of information.

From such studies, one might infer both that data content is more important than data frequency or quantity, and that the level of summary or detail depends on the underlying dynamics of the clinical and financial processes being managed. When such processes are predictable and fairly static, without too much variability, summary data are best; however, if processes are unpredictable and dynamic, more detailed data are necessary for effective decision making.

The Right Person at the Right Time

Information should be supplied only when action is possible and necessary. If data and analyses are presented only when requested, many routine reports can be discontinued.[18,19]

Research has shown that a beneficial relationship exists between use of information systems and effective manager or professional performance.[20] A manager or clinician who has a positive attitude toward computer information systems and a records-orientation management style (that is, a tendency to keep records) can improve performance through use of information support systems.

Getting the right data to the right person at the right time depends to a large degree on the decision style of the managers, executives, and clinicians involved. Consequently, the most effective information support system provides each manager, executive, and clinician access to his or her own selected data indicators on individualized time cycles. The key to success lies in using the technology of decision support systems and executive information systems, making easy-to-use data access languages available, making data widely available, providing staff to teach and assist with its use, and promoting individualized access.

The Future of Data as a Resource

In the future, all access to comprehensive information may be performed through computer technology. Steady and dramatic increases both in the capability of computer technology and in the extent of human knowledge have resulted in exponentially growing repositories of data. Today, data are often still stored in isolated data files, where they are incomplete and possibly misleading in the absence of synthesizing information technology. But information technology is now becoming available to provide the necessary synthesizing effect.

Gaining Insight through Advanced Uses of Data

In the new market-driven health care environment, information will be necessary to convince price-conscious health care buyers that they are receiving value for their dollars. A health care institution's computerized data base and information support system can provide the data resources and analytical capability necessary to achieve this goal.

An important opportunity can be found in innovative statistical analysis techniques that identify a health care institution's performance strengths and weaknesses. Simple statistical analyses of transactions such as patterns of patient transfers among rooms, for example, could identify service logjams and delays during patients' stays. Also, statistical analyses of new patient encounters, demographics, and geographic data could identify unanticipated trends in patient referral and admission patterns. And, finally, correlation analysis can provide insight into some important outcomes otherwise unmeasurable: for example, statistical analysis of patient acuity data correlated with socioeconomic status could detect patterns of patients' compliancy with prescribed medical regimens (such as medication administration instructions), possibly indicating that special intervention services should be offered to selected patients to ensure desirable outcomes and to reduce length of stay or likelihood of readmission for the same or a related problem.

Another opportunity lies in providing a means to select future courses of action by using the institution's data base and computer technology to analyze alternative plans and strategies. For example, computer modeling might be used in "what if" analyses to test the outcome of future pricing or marketing strategies.

Knowledge-Based Systems

Knowledge-based systems introduce the prospect of computers that perform at a level comparable to intelligent human behavior. Knowledge-based systems (or *expert systems,* as they are also called) require that a set of rules be stored in the computer along with raw data. Together, the stored rules and data transform a data base into a knowledge base.

Knowledge-based systems routinely apply defined rules to data and, by reasoning in an automated way, draw logical inferences. Rules are obtained by first capturing the approaches and decision trees of experts in a field and then declaring those rules to the computer. These declared rules guide the system through a series of if-then logic steps, emulating the logic paths that an expert would follow when solving a particular problem. Such an automated system not only makes expertise available to less-experienced people, but also can be used to help the experts themselves by relieving them of routine work and allowing them to concentrate on exceptions.

Knowledge-based systems are used in the insurance business, for example, to help make insurance underwriting decisions and to determine the amount of premium to charge. In health care, a knowledge-based system called INTERNIST has been developed experimentally for diagnosing illnesses, using step-by-step rules that simulate physicians' thought processes. Such systems are also being used in instructional processes in medical schools and teaching hospitals.

Knowledge-based systems will be best used in health care to determine courses of action that depend on existing conditions in situations where criteria for the decisions can be declared and the data can be made available. They will eventually be used in many processes in health care: in quality assurance, for choosing patient charts to audit, or in internal auditing, for choosing departmental processes to audit. They may also be used to sense details necessary to prepare discharge plans, such as sensing age, marital status, living arrangements, and diagnosis, as well as test results, diet requirements, and medications prescribed. Similarly, they may also be used to prescribe nursing care plans. They may also be used to accept signals from medical instruments, analyze them together with other data, and, when necessary, alert medical personnel of possible problems. They could ultimately perform many checklist activities throughout the work of a health care institution, anywhere the system can compare data and recorded activities against a script of what should occur and against normal ranges of values of outcomes, alerting personnel of the institution whenever conditions deviate from those expected.

The Future: Exploiting Data to Extend Human Capability

Knowledge-based computer information systems will eventually supplement human thought processes in health care. As more and more of the medical record is stored in computer data bases, future information support systems will be used in a wide range of computer applications to provide medical alerts and diagnostic reminders, to monitor exceptions from norms, and to support management and clinical decisions in a myriad of new ways. Human minds create ideas, but comprehensive data bases and advanced computer information systems will be used to shape the information that fuels those ideas.

Notes

1. K. Matta, "Impact of Prospective Pricing on the Information System in the Health Care Industry," *Journal of Medical Systems* 12, no. 1 (1988): 57–66.
2. N. M. Lorenzi and E. B. Marks, "University of Cincinnati Medical Center: Integrating Information," *Bulletin of the Medical Library Association* 76, no. 3 (July 1988): 231–36.
3. P. Ein-Dor and E. Segev, *A Paradigm for Management Information Systems* (New York: Praeger Publishers, 1981), p. 104.
4. Ibid., p. 175.
5. J. F. Rockart and C. V. Bullen, eds., *The Rise of Managerial Computing* (Homewood, IL: Dow Jones–Irwin, 1986), pp. 51–52.
6. Ibid., pp. 257–79, 383–423.
7. Ein-Dor and Segev, *A Paradigm,* pp. 204–5.
8. Rockart and Bullen, *The Rise of Managerial Computing,* pp. 198–99.
9. Ein-Dor and Segev, *A Paradigm,* p. 118.
10. F. W. McFarlan and J. L. McKenney, *Corporate Information Systems Management: The Issues Facing Senior Executives* (Homewood, IL: Richard D. Irwin, Inc., 1983), pp. 41–48.

11. Rockart and Bullen, *The Rise of Managerial Computing,* p. 261.
12. Ibid.
13. Ein-Dor and Segev, *A Paradigm,* p. 176.
14. Rockart and Bullen, *The Rise of Managerial Computing,* pp. 210–23.
15. Ein-Dor and Segev, *A Paradigm,* pp. 106–8.
16. Ibid., p. 113.
17. Ibid., pp. 110–11.
18. Ibid., p. 105.
19. Ibid., p. 117.
20. Ibid., pp. 191–94.

10

LOOKING AHEAD: INFORMATION TECHNOLOGY AND DRAMATIC IMPROVEMENTS IN HEALTH CARE

Many industries have harnessed information technology advances to power dramatic improvements in productivity and products. Thus far, however, many factors have inhibited the advanced use of information technology in health care. The labor-intensive, hands-on nature of health care delivery, the life-or-death consequences of mistakes, and the medical and nursing professions' ingrained procedural traditions have all served as barriers to change.

Many other factors, however, are now beginning to prompt considerable advancements in the use of information technology in health care. Skyrocketing costs, shrinking reimbursement, quality-of-care issues, nursing shortages, competition among hospitals, and increased public scrutiny are creating pressure for managed change. The labor-intensive nature of health care is a force in itself, providing a multitude of opportunities to improve productivity and quality while reducing costs through use of information technology. The information-intensive nature of health care also offers numerous opportunities for information technology use. Meanwhile, information technology's reliability and capability are rapidly improving, and computer equipment costs are decreasing. In particular, networking and end-user computing are improving at a rapid pace, and these are precisely the technologies promising the data-sharing and work-sharing capabilities that can contribute most to increased productivity in an information- and labor-intensive industry.

Clinical and other professional users, who at one time were skeptical and unenthusiastic about computers, are now beginning to perceive the technology as practical and valuable. These clinicians are another force driving health care institutions to enthusiastically embrace the use of information technology.

These powerful forces, combined with good planning and management, can transform today's problems and opportunities into tomorrow's dramatic improvements in health care practice and management.

Doing Business Electronically

Consider the possibility of modems that handle integrated voice, data, images, and text, connecting people and information sources throughout the health care industry within a few seconds. Visualize the potential of telecommunications that eliminate time constraints from clinical and financial transactions. Ponder the almost limitless value of efficient information linkages among people that share data and work. Far from being fantasy, these technological opportunities are almost upon us.

In *Competitive Advantage: Creating and Sustaining Superior Performance,* Michael Porter suggests that the successful institutions of the future will be those that achieve a "sustainable competitive advantage" by managing tightly controlled work linkages in a "value chain."[1] An institution's value chain is the sequence of linked work that results in a finished product; success is achieved by efficiently managing the chain of integrated work processes. Porter predicts a changed management structure in the future, one that will use information systems technology to make the value chain as tightly connected and efficient as possible. With information technology, management's focus will shift from managing work activities to managing linkages among work activities.

Advanced computer communications technology will provide a powerful strategic tool to the health care industry. It will create new information channels within each health care institution and across the external boundaries of institutions. It will offer automation opportunities to improve procedures, controls, information sharing, and working procedures among groups as diverse as physicians and suppliers of materials and supplies.

Gaining Productivity through Networking

Advanced computer communications technology will spark a shift in emphasis from management of a clinical department to management of work activities and work relationships among several departments. For example, orders and services among departments may be managed through computerized work lists and work scheduling among departments. This may be the most promising productivity-enhancing opportunity available to health care institutions.

Continued changes in health care will exert escalating pressures for improved productivity. And, in the labor-intensive clinical work of health care, it makes sense to invest in information technology that increases clinicians' productivity. Institutions will significantly improve the performance of clinicians by using information technology that enhances the efficiency of human interaction. Computer networks will allow data to be transferred or indirectly shared among people who are working on partitioned parts of the same patient case or other hospital project. Moreover, clinicians and other knowledge workers will save time by using electronic mail to communicate quickly and efficiently.

Information technology will also enhance work activities that cross departmental boundaries. Networks linking physicians, nurses, and clinical departments will improve work efficiencies and work quality among diverse clinical groups, strengthen controls, and focus more quickly and more clearly on problems. These same networks will help clinicians gain the immediate attention of other clinicians, thereby eliminating delays that would otherwise inevitably occur.

Networking technology, along with the immediate access it affords, will help to promote more specialization by institutional specialists by making their expertise more available to others through networks, and will therefore tend to promote their increased presence in health care institutions. Specialists' participation in cooperative work will be improved through networking and electronic mail, and they will apply their expertise through the network by sending information and messages or by actually contributing to shared work. As specialists become more available, institutions will become more dependent on them—and departments will be less likely to develop separate expertise in the specialists' fields. Thus, advanced capabilities for networking, and the accompanying information flow, will tend to move organizations toward a higher level of teamwork among specialists.

As a result of the effects of computer communications technology, computers will also alter the nature of work relationships both among workers and between workers and management. Managers and coordinators of work will communicate work schedules and work status through networks, such as the daily calendaring of meetings that is already occurring in some organizations. Furthermore, computerized usage logs can be used to record and monitor a myriad of worker performance indicators: number of transactions performed per day (for example, number of orders entered) response times between one department's request and another department's response (for example, how much time was required to clean and make available a

patient room following the previous patient's discharge), average time between the steps of an automated sequence (for example, how much time was
required for video workstation users to think and judge between work steps),
and the time each day that personnel spend working at their video workstations. As this type of record keeping becomes more widely used, management will be required to sensitively select performance monitoring methods
that are effective but that are not perceived as invasions of privacy.

Computerized Business Relationships beyond the Walls

Computer communications linkages will enable health care institutions to
tightly manage their value chain even across external boundaries. Useful
electronic connections and alliances can be forged among health care institutions, physicians, suppliers, payers, and patients, all of whom have an interest in improving the cost effectiveness of health care.

Strategic hospital-physician relationships

One of the most important health care work linkages exists between physicians and hospital data in patients' charts and medical records. Tomorrow's
health care setting may allow patient care to be given in any of several
alternative physical settings, possibly including patient care in the patient's
home, provided by a physician from his or her home. The value chain toward
high-quality patient care under these conditions will be extremely difficult
to maintain without high-quality data links that extend beyond the walls of
buildings and institutions.

With computer communications connections to hospital information
systems, physicians can use video computer terminals to gain immediate
access to rounds lists, pertinent information about patients' medical conditions, status of orders and results, and other reference sources that the hospital could provide, such as library bibliographic sources and drug reference
information. Computerized access to the hospital's information system provides physicians with immediate and same-day access to outpatient test results, allowing more rapid diagnosis and treatment and also eliminating the
need to telephone hospital labs repeatedly in order to obtain test results. Such
access could conceivably lower physicians' staff expenses, ultimately reducing the cost to patients.

Physicians who can access patient data from computers in their homes
have reported that such access gives them an opportunity to review and
evaluate data, and make important patient treatment decisions in a nonpres-
sured environment. One physician reported that this kind of access provides

him "more time to explore possible explanations and to think about how to proceed with the patient's care."[2]

From such computerized linkages, physician office staff could gain access to financial data required for patient billing. For example, when a patient is referred to a physician for consultation, the office to which the patient is being referred might not otherwise have necessary insurance information about that patient.

Similarly, a physician who is called in to consult on a case could access patient data directly from his or her office as soon as the consult is requested, allowing for thorough preparation for the case even before the patient is seen. And future computerized linkages could facilitate referrals and physician-to-physician messages via a form of electronic mail.

Of course, computerized linkages with physicians can generate yet another benefit. By helping a health care institution build closer working relationships with physicians, such linkages could increase the probability that physicians will admit their patients to its hospital. Physicians might prefer to admit patients to a hospital that has invested in computerized linkages that improve the efficiency of their work and the quality of health care.

Sharing information and services with other hospitals

Computerized linkages can also be useful in providing record keeping that serves the common needs of several hospitals. When a hospital provides other hospitals with service for calibration and maintenance of biomedical instruments, for example, a computer communications linkage might be used to track equipment that is scheduled for inspection or other attention, where the equipment is physically located, the contact person who arranges for servicing, and service records. Both hospitals could gain access to the data base: one to check schedules and enter the results of work, and the other to verify completion and to retrieve data about repair records. A similar kind of linkage could also allow one hospital to order materials from the warehouse of another hospital.

Hospitals that routinely transfer patients to other facilities for additional care or aftercare could also effectively utilize computerized linkages to share patient data. Institutions sharing computerized data bases of diagnostic and treatment information are able to provide better continuity of care.

As mergers and acquisitions increasingly occur in the health care industry, computerized linkages among hospitals could become a necessity. A merger of two hospitals might require that employees and physicians work in both hospitals, creating strong incentive for establishing a computerized linkage among the two institutions' computer information systems. Such a linkage not only makes patient data available for continuity of patient care, but also requires employees and physicians to understand and use only one common computer information system, regardless of the hospital facility in which they work.

Linkages with suppliers

Porter argues that the value chain's efficiency can be significantly enhanced by building strong electronic linkages with suppliers. Direct access to suppliers' merchandise catalogs can be achieved through electronic linkages, and desired items can then be ordered directly. Such a system eliminates time-consuming phone calls and paperwork, while also accelerating delivery of ordered items. Merchandise is consequently available more rapidly, allowing health care institutions to save further by reducing investment in inventory. Large inventories will become obsolete when needed supplies can be quickly obtained from suppliers.

Linkages with payers

Electronic linkages with payers will soon replace the practice of mailing claims in paper form. Such a process will reduce paperwork and, therefore, save clerical work time, accelerate reimbursement, speed up cash flow, and increase working capital.

Linkages with patients

A new telecommunications industry service called Integrated Services Digital Network (ISDN) is becoming available. This digital communications service, made available much like conventional voice telephone service is made available, will provide inexpensive, high-speed, high-quality data communications linkages similar to voice communication. ISDN will allow patients in their homes to access a network and transmit data to another location, such as to a hospital's computerized diagnostic equipment. Alternatively, monitoring equipment in the patient's home could be connected to a health care institution for interpretation by a clinician or for calibration by an authorized technician.

    The computer communications service, used in tandem with technology that stores important patient data on a wallet-sized card, could be made available through computer linkages between patients and remote sites with which they are connected for diagnosis. Results of diagnosis or treatment could then be transmitted and stored on the card along with the patient health history already stored there.

Developing Necessary Data Exchange Standards

For computer communications technology and related future instrumentation and recording devices to be truly effective, universal standards must exist so that these various devices can exchange data with one another. Typically, equipment and software developed by different vendors have different data and processing characteristics, just as different languages use different alphabets and rules of syntax.

To solve this problem, a prominent international professional society, the Institute of Electrical and Electronics Engineers (IEEE), has established a special committee to study alternatives and to declare standards. The committee is called MEDIX (Medical Data Exchange); their multiyear project has been christened IEEE Standards Project #1157. The effort's stated objective is "to specify and establish a robust and flexible communications standard for the exchange of data between heterogeneous healthcare information systems."[3] Already, the product of this important work is emerging and has affected the design of computer systems produced during 1990.

Information Technology that Supports
Patient Care Directly

In the not-too-distant future, computer technology will be used to assist in the management of clinical outcomes. Faced with capped revenues and rising costs, health care institutions have no choice but to apply computer technology more directly to patient care in their struggle to contain costs while maintaining high quality of care. We are clearly entering an era during which the progress of a patient's care will be more closely monitored and managed, and computer technology will provide opportunities to manage patient care cost and quality more effectively. Future systems will be designed to focus on step-by-step monitoring of care and to provide more direct support for the work of clinicians.

Integrating Medical Instrumentation Data

For some time, vendors of clinical diagnostic and patient monitoring equipment have been providing valuable new medical instruments that typically feature some embedded computer technology. Data provided by these computerized medical instruments are usually displayed on video and printing consoles but, unfortunately, have not been automatically integrated with results from other instruments and aggregated in medical data bases. Consequently, such data are not used as thoroughly as they could be, resulting in ambiguities, delays, and inefficiencies in patient care. Although great strides have been made in efforts to enhance these instruments' capabilities, an increasing number of clerical transcribing tasks are required to utilize the resulting data. In the advanced medical instruments systems of the future, data will be funneled directly into integrated patient care data bases. The availability of accumulated and consolidated data will allow retrieval of test results together with other related data in the data bases, thereby improving the productivity of the clinical personnel and the quality of diagnostic and treatment processes.

Aggregated Computerized Medical Records

Aggregated data in future data bases will provide a valuable resource for management of both institutions and patient care. Although the concept of managing data as a special institutional resource is relatively new, health care institutions will be able to manage their data resources effectively by defining hospitalwide data dictionaries and implementing technology that integrates the data bases of distributed computers.

Data bases will also be used to sense and track relevant information embedded in that data. Such data will not only be used directly in the administration of patient care, but will also be used retrospectively to detect physicians' diagnostic and treatment protocols in use, outliers, and trends.

Data bases will not only provide direct support of patient care, but they will also indirectly support preventive medicine by providing information, under appropriate confidentiality controls, for research and analysis. This use of data for research and analysis promises great opportunities for reducing the cost of health care over the long term.

Knowledge-Based Systems

Knowledge-based systems, using stored data and defined rules to mimic the mental processes of experts, will become increasingly useful in improving quality and consistency of health care in the future.[4] They will help improve productivity by allowing caregivers to select the best choice from among a broad and complex range of diagnostic and treatment options. They will help monitor test results, vital signs, and other clinical indicators to see if they are out of the normal range or off the normal track, and be able to signal alerts when a higher level of expertise must be brought to bear on a medical problem. Knowledge-based systems will complement, not replace, the traditional work of clinicians. Academic interest will be attracted to these systems, and venture capitalists will seek entrepreneurial opportunities to invest in knowledge-based systems that support clinical decisions. Computer technology will never replace human capacity for creative thought, but knowledge-based systems will liberate clinical personnel to apply their intelligence more effectively and selectively. Faster, more capable large computers and progressively powerful desktop workstations will support growth in knowledge-based systems' contributions to the work of people.

Improved Computer-Human Interfaces

As computer-mediated processes are extended to people beyond institutional walls, the technology must inevitably be made easier to use. Health care institutions cannot expect physicians and patients to tolerate the same awkwardness and difficulties that were imposed on clerical and administrative personnel as their work was automated in computer systems of the past. Standards and conventions for use of keyboards will be established, even among the products of several vendors. Pointing devices will be embedded in the video terminal technology. Error messages will be more understandable. Computerized instructional help will be easily available. Workstations will display high-resolution images, and wallet-sized cards on which data are recorded will become an integral part of the new environment.

The computer's potential for graphics will also greatly improve. Even now, computers are being used to display objects in three dimensions, with the added capability of rotating these images. Physicians, following the lead of architects and engineers, will harness computer graphics processing to create high-resolution graphics of the human anatomy. Medical treatment will be planned by viewing graphics of the human body on video screens, and the images will be rotated and magnified to provide many perspectives. Images will also be superimposed on each other, just as nightly TV weather presentations superimpose states' geographical boundaries on video versions of satellite weather maps. Graphics technology will also employ computer power to analyze the images, using complex mathematical analysis to potentially interpret subtle distinctions that the human eye is unable to detect.

Storage and Retrieval of New Types of Data

Optical disk storage, a new type of data storage medium, will allow greater capabilities for storing information. During the 30-year history of computing technology, there were traditionally only two types of media for permanent storage of computer data: magnetic tape and magnetic disk storage. Now, optical disk storage has emerged as an alternative capable of storing much more data at much lower cost. With this increased capability, data in the form of image and voice records will soon be stored as easily as text and numerical data have been stored in the past.

Digital imaging

The future will offer information in image form that is digitized, stored, and integrated with text and numerical data in the patient's computerized medical record. These images will be retrievable along with other data.

Diagnostic images, such as those produced by radiology and cardiology imaging equipment, will be collected and stored in digitized form. Optical disk storage devices will permit large volumes of images to be inexpensively stored, and retrieval of these images will be both simple (using indexing methods such as medical record number), and direct (without requiring physical retrieval from archival storage in a remote storeroom). The images will be transmitted across high-speed optical networks to nursing stations, clinics, and physicians' offices, where high-resolution monitors will display them on desktop workstations for quick reference during the administration of patient care.

Other work documents from the patient's chart will also be stored in image form. Face sheets, nursing notes, and other paper documents will be scanned by computerized scanning equipment and stored on inexpensive disk storage, instead of on microfilm or microfiche. Storage of images in this manner will reduce costs, require fewer clerical personnel, provide better access, allow easier searching, and provide technological features such as magnification and windowing of one document on top of another. Storing digitized images of text documents will prove more useful than transcribing the written material into text because image scanning preserves all information appearing on the original: notes in margins, handwritten underlines for emphasis, deletion marks, and other handwritten annotations.

Storing voice recordings

Voice messages will also eventually be stored in digital form. The several stored forms of information—text, data, images, and voice—will be integrated together in data base records and will be available for retrieval together or separately.

Computer Technology at the Point-of-Care

For nursing personnel, the task of charting is a labor-intensive and intellectually draining task that will be displaced, to a great extent, by computer technology. The best nurses will choose to work where the best productivity-enhancing and care-enhancing tools are available, and point-of-care data-recording and data-retrieval mechanisms will provide those tools.

Physicians also will value comprehensive information technology that brings relevant information quickly to bear on patient care. Such technology puts accurate information at their fingertips and ensures better and more efficient diagnosis and treatment.

Providing nursing support

Advanced computer technology will establish nursing stations as the hub of a future computerized nursing information system. This nursing information system will support nursing personnel directly, as well as supporting patient care in general like today's hospital information systems. It will serve as the repository for an aggregation of clinical information that will benefit both nurses and physicians in providing patient care. Various members of the care-giving team will bear responsibility for creating and maintaining the clinical information that contributes to the nursing information system's data base. Nursing personnel will likely accept primary information collection and recording tasks because they will anticipate a payoff of saved time, increased productivity, and improved quality of patient care. In contrast, today's hospital information systems require much work from nursing personnel and offer little value to them in return.

Bedside or portable data collection equipment will gather data from patient monitors. Vital signs will be collected and recorded electronically. In addition, hand-held bar code readers will be used at the bedside to record medication administration. Display equipment, such as high-resolution video displays and advanced laser printers, will display and print data using formats resembling those currently used, but they will also allow new and innovative variations, such as showing several different measured trends on the same graphic display. The resulting clinical data repository will contribute significantly to the computerized medical record of the future.

Nursing information systems will also provide the means for recording nursing diagnosis, severity of illness, and intensity of nursing care. This and other recorded data about patients' conditions will be accessed by knowledge-based systems that will recommend nursing care plans and discharge plans.

The data repository will likely be known as the nursing information system (instead of hospital information system, patient data management system, or some other name), acknowledging that data are collected, maintained, and managed primarily by nursing personnel. This new focus will provide the catalyst for a long-overdue shift in nursing documentation and nursing procedures. It will reduce the time, effort, and expense currently spent on paperwork; it may also lead to greater professional prestige by emphasizing the importance of nursing diagnosis and nursing care planning, as opposed to the current dominance of care planning that depends almost solely on physician diagnosis. Such recognition could additionally motivate nursing personnel to contribute more significantly to the advancement of the use of computer technology in health care. Such systems will also serve as a valuable nurse recruitment asset in those institutions that are able to successfully define, implement, and manage advanced nursing information systems.

Providing physician support

Physicians and their office staffs can look forward to increased dependence on computer terminals for access to clinical data. Personnel in physicians' offices will access patient data through their office computers, eliminating the inefficiencies and delays of telephone calls to various hospital departments for patient test results. They will also rely on computer access to acquire information about services offered by health care institutions, referencing catalogs of information about diagnostic services provided by different service departments, and to inquire about necessary scheduling and preparation. Instead of telephoning the hospital, for example, they will enter orders and schedule tests and treatment directly from their computer terminals.

When physicians become comfortable using computers, they will expect to access additional information through computer workstations. They will use their workstations to gain quick access to up-to-date drug reference information, bibliographic information from libraries, information from the nursing information system, and text data such as, for example, medical staff bylaws and hospital protocols for determination of death. Eventually, physicians will rely on computerized access to data just as they now depend on patient charts at nursing stations—and they will expect such access to be available from computer workstations at nursing stations, in other areas of the hospital, in their offices, and even in their homes.

Supporting Patient Care Management

The aggregation of all patient care data will ultimately comprise a computerized medical record that serves as the reference point for management of clinical outcomes. In addition to other justifications for comprehensive record keeping, managed care programs such as HMOs and PPOs will force hospitals to develop effective record-keeping systems in order to ensure adequate pricing.

Aggregated data will be invaluable in analyzing information to establish pricing of contracts. It will also help hospitals respond efficiently to employers' requests for summarized data on their employees' use and costs of services. It will allow the hospital to track specific cases and groups of cases and to identify the differences between the best cases, in terms of quality and cost, and the worst cases, possibly identifying causes and effects of each. Readmission and continuity of care data will also be available for episode-to-episode analysis. And some of this data may be summarized and presented in the executive information systems of the future, enabling management to take quick and effective action based on the insight gained.

Managing Complex New Work Relationships

Advanced information technology will provide solutions to hospital problems and provide opportunities for competitive advantage, but its implementation will tax the skills of health care executives who must face the decision of when to use it and for what purposes. It will also tax the management savvy of those who must manage the institutional change that such technology will bring. And it will tax the management skills of those who must manage its use as it brings added complexity to the work of people throughout the health care institution.

As information technology such as networking, distributed computing, and large shared data bases come into wide use, the physical work of the health care institution will change dramatically. For example, work will become more abstract. The results of work performed at a computer workstation are not easily observable and measurable by departmental supervisors, unlike bundles of paper or other physical work products. Computer systems will make it more difficult for a supervisor to determine where work is being performed or neglected. It will also be more difficult to quickly place accountability for work poorly performed or left undone. Consequently, new methods must be put in place to manage the interdependencies among the work of many departments.

Executive management will be required to face three new challenges as computers generate increasingly interdependent work in institutions:

1. The challenge of planning and managing institutional change as information technology becomes a basic necessity and transforms the institution's internal structure, affecting roles, resources, power, and hierarchy

2. The challenge of managing interdependence among partitioned parts of the institution's work as departmental and institutional boundaries blur, with work performed by team-based, problem-focused, frequently changing groups that are in turn supported by computers and computerized communications

3. The challenge of managing the implementation, operation, and use of information technology resources

Managing Institutional Resources and Change

Vast numbers of jobs will be automated during the next few years as information technology becomes a basic need of institutions. Some changes will be welcomed by the physicians and hospital personnel involved; some will be resisted. Some changes will strengthen the hospital's productivity; some potentially could weaken it. Because uncertainty of value and success is inherent in most information technology projects, enthusiasm for change will be countered by conservatism. Departments and people have established beliefs and norms in their work environments. Efforts to implement automation in that work culture consequently will be difficult and, to be successful, must be managed with consummate skill.

Because only innovative and decisive health care institutions will reap the full rewards of advanced information technology, management must identify opportunities for change, make change happen, take advantage of change, and sustain change, in order to benefit from its potential. Information technology essential to health care will advance continuously, so health care institutions must also change continuously, always searching for new ways to improve processes and, therefore, performance. Both health care organizations and their computer information systems will be in a constant state of change, requiring that comprehensive training and retraining be consistently available to both support and sustain valued change.

The key to managing change is to make sophisticated use of leadership skills. Change must be planned and communicated, and consensus must be gained. Broad-based project teams must be engaged. Sensitive team leaders must stimulate innovative thinking and cohesive action while also imposing controls, ultimately leading to a delicate balance of innovative risks and prudent precautions.

Managing Interdependent Work

Although the need to manage interdependence among the work of many is not new, it will be in the forefront of productivity issues facing health care institutions' senior management in the future. Recent literature suggests that one of information technology's most important roles in tomorrow's institutions will be providing new approaches to managing complex organizational interdependence.[5]

Information technology's impact on people and organizations will be caused by both the continuing widespread use of the technology for direct productivity enhancements, and by the use of information technology capabilities to help manage complex organizational work. For example, computer systems now in use improve the productivity of workers, but are already making work more abstract and blurring partitions among the work of different departments, eroding the efficiency of interdepartmental work. At the same time, health care industry pressures require that the work of many departments be made more efficient.

One driving force leading to increasingly interdependent work is the convergence of several computer-related technologies: traditional computing, data communication, office automation, and medical instrumentation. This convergence will spur yet more data communications advances, which will in turn reinforce the movement toward interdependent work. Another force driving institutions inexorably to interdependent work can be found in the work force's rising expectations: workers have simply come to expect easy access to information they need to perform their jobs.

Nevertheless, the journey toward interdependent work should progress a bit more smoothly in health care than in other industries. In fact, traditional working relationships in health care institutions may be well suited to the use of advanced computer information systems for the sharing of work. The work of patient care has historically been performed through firmly established, cooperative working relationships among health care professionals, whereas other industries rely on distinctly hierarchical working relationships. Consequently, health care institutions should more readily adapt to, and benefit from, modern information technology.

Information technology can be used in many ways to make the cooperative work of health care professionals even more efficient: to share and exchange data, to generate interdepartmental work lists automatically, and to sense and alert higher levels of clinicians or management when conditions warrant. The technology can reduce imprecision in coordinated activity among people, helping them choose the right path among many alternatives.

However, information technology's power should not be overzealously exploited to the point where automated record keeping of worker activity exceeds requirements for management of interdepartmental work. Management must guard against intimidating and humbling workers by imposing productivity standards based on the numbers of and timing of computer transactions performed. Attempting to wring additional productivity out of the work force by means of computerized espionage on worker activity will simply add unnecessary additional stress to already stressful jobs.

Management must also guard against drawing health care personnel into a crippling obsession with computer technology, which can lead to long hours of work at night and possibly cause fatigue, skeletal problems, eyestrain, and other health problems. Personnel who adopt such an increasingly stressful work pattern eventually burn out.[6]

Finally, considering the interdependent work of the two broad groups involved—computer professionals and clinical and departmental computer users—management must also invest substantial effort in overcoming the legacy of competition, criticism, and hostility that has traditionally existed between the two groups. The relationships must instead be transformed into a focused and cooperative team effort.

Managing Implementation and Use of Information Technology

The overwhelming complexity of future technological alternatives will pose significant management problems. Health care institutions must be able to accurately assess information technology's capabilities and limitations in order to formulate sound technical and management decisions. Management will be forced to keep abreast of technological advancements continuing at a fast pace in telecommunications, networking, end-user computing, decision support systems and executive support systems, laser printing, image processing, office systems technology, knowledge-based systems, the computer-human interface, desktop workstations, packaged computer software, the capacity and reliability of computer hardware, industry standards, vendor relationships, and methods of implementing and managing information technology.

Today's shift of computing to desktop computers will continue, but future mainframe computers and large minicomputers will also be more powerful. Mainframe computers and large minicomputers will become progressively less visible, but they will continue to house the large data bases, to serve as the hub of networks, and to be the workhorses supporting many mainstream financial and clinical transactions. Large computers will be indispensable for processing that requires vast quantities of instantly available data. But, because computer power costs much less in a desktop computer than in a large computer, the large computers should no longer be used for any processing that can realistically be performed by desktop workstations.

Redundant, backup equipment will become increasingly prevalent and expected for all computers, telecommunications equipment, electric power, chilled water (used in air-conditioning or cooling units), and other technology in which a single failure could cripple an institution's computer capability. This redundancy could take the form of ready-to-use backup equipment; dual units sharing a processing load, each of which could function independently should one of them fail; or a behind-the-scenes second unit functioning completely redundantly and ready to take over immediately if the primary unit fails.

Although computer hardware advances will appear at a rapid pace, lagging software developments will limit available capability. For example, computer technology advances will soon provide computers with parallel processing capabilities, in contrast to conventional computers that feature only one internal processor. Conventional computers start at the beginning of a problem and work through it sequentially; parallel processors can divide complex problems into chunks and then assign tasks to several internal processors that attack the problem simultaneously. However, software that will be able to partition work and manage its simultaneous processing will be very complex and could take many years to perfect. Software development work remains on the critical path, and its development is difficult to manage. Consequently, target dates for software completion defy prediction.

Vendors' software packages must be more flexible so that health care institutions can tailor computer information systems to their specific needs and unique environment. One drawback to today's health care software packages is that they have typically been defined and designed principally by vendors, not by potential customers. Because vendors frequently presume knowledge they do not always possess, some mismatch of products to customers' needs usually occurs. And, in the interest of business profits, vendors sometimes develop software products that require the least investment of their resources. Or they choose to develop software functions aimed at seducing target audiences. Such vendor marketing orientation all too often sacrifices substance in the interest of form, resulting in products that promote glitter (such as multicolored graphs), products that falsely promise simple computer solutions to difficult management problems, or products with superficial features that divert attention from real needs. Management must therefore guard against selections inappropriately influenced by vendor marketing. In addition, health care institutions must make a concerted effort to shift the power of product definition from vendors to customers. Without such a shift, health care institutions will find themselves perpetually force-fitting all their problems and opportunities into poorly conceived vendor products.

On the other hand, the information technology industry desperately needs standards for data exchange among clinical information systems. It is in the interest of both health care institutions and vendors that standard-setting efforts, such as the MEDIX Committee of the IEEE, succeed in establishing standards for data exchange and data sharing among systems. It is also vital that vendors provide open systems, whose details are open to others' product designs so that a system is more likely to mesh with other systems to collectively meet the customer's needs.

The computer industry eventually will provide enhanced computerized tools that aid in implementation and management of computer information systems. *Computer-aided software engineering* (CASE) is the term currently used to describe a set of techniques and potential software tools that will provide orderly and effective management processes for many activities: system definition and design, system implementation, prototyping of functions and reports, software library maintenance, problem diagnosis and management, and change management. For example, enhanced computer technology ultimately will provide a much easier framework for defining the report formats, one that approaches a fill-in-the-blanks process. Video display screens and billing formats will be defined by a similar process. Another, more elusive component could be a method that allows transformation of functional specifications into computer programs without exhaustive trial-and-error programming efforts. While the need for these various components of CASE technologies is widely acknowledged, progress in the emergence and acceptance of CASE as a recognized discipline or body of technology has been slow. Consequently, selected components are successfully emerging and will likely be used as needed and justified by management, but CASE as a single cohesive technology package seems destined to suffer a long and difficult road to maturity.

Management of information technology will continue to be a complex but extremely important institutional requirement. CIOs, the executives responsible for computer technology, will be challenged with assessing current technology, discontinuities, and new alternatives in the marketplace; with defining requirements for and acquiring new technology; with recruiting, retaining, and organizing qualified personnel: with integrating and connecting systems and aggregating data from various computer systems; and with the complex task of managing the daily operations of these people and this technology.[7] Of these, however, the one issue on which failure and success will most certainly depend is integration and harmony among the health care institution's varied computer systems. The CIO must avoid dissipating resources on inflexible and incompatible systems and on marginal contributors. Management must guide selection of information technology, seize opportunities to use the technology for the institution's benefit, and prevent it from becoming an uncontrolled drain on resources.

A Marvelous but Uncertain Threshold

Computerized information services will become increasingly important to health care institutions in the coming years. And information technology's rapid development will continue to offer lucrative opportunities for financial and clinical improvements.

Consequently, successful use of advanced information technology will become a critical factor in health care institutions' survival. Failure to recognize the magnitude of change and opportunity could lead to failure. While the leading edge yields the greatest benefits, success at the leading edge is difficult to achieve and requires strong and competent leadership for making important decisions. In this arena, the executive responsible for computer systems will play an important leadership role crucial to institutional objectives.

We are on a marvelous but uncertain threshold. As we face this frontier, cautiously planning our next projects and investments in information technology, we are plagued by uncertainty about their success and potential contributions to institutional goals and objectives. Even when a successful project improves productivity or quality of care, we cannot always be sure it lies along a path heading in the proper long-term direction.

Available financial resources are so limited, and the tolerance of employees and medical staff so precious, that these assets cannot be wasted on projects that offer only the glitter of new gadgetry that cannot become part of an integrated total system. Time and effort must be invested in understanding the technology, some of it mature and some very primitive. Plans and objectives must be communicated to the diverse populations within our health care institutions. We must plan information technology extensions and then successfully manage their implementation and use.

Considering the current business climate in health care—and forecasts of stormier times yet to come—we can no longer tolerate credibility-eroding project failures or the disharmony generated by poorly selected, false solutions. We cannot let ourselves be held hostage by vendors, cults, fads, or the empire-building mentalities of individual hospital departments. We can do better.

Notes

1. M. E. Porter, *Competitive Advantage: Creating and Sustaining Superior Performance* (New York: The Free Press, 1985), p. 50.
2. "Linking Up with the Future of Medicine," *Medical Staff*, The Methodist Hospital, Houston, Texas, 6, no. 2 (March 1989): 1, 3–4.
3. Institute of Electrical and Electronics Engineers, Medical Data Interchange

Committee, IEEE Standards Project #1157, MEDIX, minutes of September 7, 1988, meeting.

4. E. Pollack, "Expert Systems: Fact or Fantasy?" *Computers in Healthcare* (December 1989): 31–37.

5. J. F. Rockart and J. E. Short, "IT in the 1990s: Managing Organizational Interdependence," *Sloan Management Review* (Winter 1989): 7–17.

6. P. H. Lewis, "When Machines Spawn Obsession," *New York Times,* November 13, 1988, p. F-9.

7. J. J. Donovan, "Beyond Chief Information Officer to Network Manager," *Harvard Business Review* 66, no. 5 (September–October 1988): 134–40.

GLOSSARY

This glossary contains terms used in the text as well as terms that are often used in discussing current issues in planning, selecting, implementing, and managing information technology.

Acceptance Test. The test of computer system software or hardware after implementation to ensure that the requirements are met. *See also* Debug; Parallel Test.

Access Control. Management and technological methods used to ensure that a computer system, including its software and data, can be accessed only by authorized users in authorized ways.

Application Package. *See* Application Software.

Application Program. A computer program that performs work for a user, such as a program that performs patient registration functions.

Application Software. A collection of application programs designed to serve a specific set of requirements (an application).

Application System. *See* Application Software.

Application Systems Plan. A list of all application systems projects under way and planned, including project descriptions, justifications, priorities, dependencies among projects, and estimated level of resources required.

Application Systems Portfolio. The collection of all the application systems of an institution.

Archiving. The systematic unloading of data from a computer system's active files to a storage medium from which the data can be later retrieved and reloaded into the active files if necessary.

Artificial Intelligence. The capability of a computer system to perform functions that are normally considered to require the intelligence of humans, such as reasoning and learning. *See also* Expert System.

Asynchronous (ASYNC). A term usually used to describe data communications among computers, in which the exchange is not synchronized. An early method of computer-to-computer communications, generally used for fairly simple connections operating at slower data communications speeds. *Contrast with* Synchronous.

Audit. To review and examine the activities of a computer information system to test the adequacy and effectiveness of procedures for data security and data integrity. *See also* Log.

Audit Trail. A step-by-step recording of the path of important steps of the processing of transactions through a computer system.

Automatic Call-Back Unit. A dialing device that permits a computer to automatically dial return calls to remote computers requesting access, to verify authorization, and to make connections among computers.

Backbone Network. In a local area network, a high-speed portion of the network to which network units and slower and smaller local networks are connected. *See also* Local Area Network.

Backup. A file or complete computer system that can be used in the event of a malfunction.

Backup Copy. A copy, usually of a file, that is kept in case the original is unintentionally changed or destroyed.

Bar Code. A code representing characters by sets of parallel bars of varying thickness and separation. Bar codes are usually printed on small labels that are placed on items of inventory (or even people) to identify them. Bar codes are read by bar code readers.

Bar Code Reader. A device that is used to scan bar codes and read them into the memory of a computer system. *See also* Bar Code.

BASIC. The acronym for Beginner's All-Purpose Symbolic Instruction Code, a high-level computer programming language with a small number of statements and a simple syntax. It is designed to be easily learned and is widely used for computer programming on microcomputers. *See also* Computer Language.

Batch Processing. A method of computer processing in which data items are grouped together for processing as a unit.

Baud Rate. A term used to refer to speed of data communication, in bits per second. For example, if the baud rate for a communication link is 2,400 baud, this means that data are being transmitted at the rate of 2,400 bits per second, approximately 300 characters (or bytes) per second.

Bit. Abbreviation for binary digit. One binary digit, either the number 1 or the number 0. *See also* Byte.

Boot. To prepare a computer system for operation by loading an operating system. *See also* Operating System.

Bridge. *See* Network Bridge.

Bug. An inadvertent mistake made by a computer programmer in writing the logic of a computer program.

Bus. Inside a computer, the physical electronic circuitry over which data are internally transferred among the internal portions of the computer, such as from and to memory and from and to its video display unit.

Byte. A set of eight adjacent binary digits (bits) that can be used to represent one alphabetic character (that is, A through Z) or one numeric character (that is, 1 through 9) or one special character (for example, $, !, ?, *). *See also* Bit; Character.

Cathode Ray Tube (CRT). A device similar to a television screen upon which data can be displayed by a computer.

CD-ROM. A compact disk used for high-capacity read-only memory, using optical media.

Central Processing Unit (CPU). The portion of a computer system that contains the circuits that execute the computer instructions.

Character. A letter, digit, or punctuation mark used in a computer system. One character is represented by a binary code composed of eight bits and is also referred to as a byte. *See also* Bit; Byte.

Chief Information Officer (CIO). The executive responsible for computer information systems and services.

Chip. A powerful unit of electronic computer technology, equivalent to many thousands of transistors, etched on a very small surface, usually of silicon.

CIO. *See* Chief Information Officer.

Client/Server Processing. *See* Cooperative Processing.

Clinical (or Medical) Information System. A computer information system that supports patient care activities, such as recording of orders and results in diagnostic and treatment departments.

Coaxial Cable. A cable consisting of one conductor, usually a small copper wire, within and insulated from another conductor of larger diameter, usually braided copper wire.

COBOL (Common Business-Oriented Language). A computer language used in programming business computer systems. The statements of COBOL resemble the English language, so this language allows fairly easy communication among individuals who must work together on a computer programming project. *See also* Computer Language.

Communication Link. The physical means of connecting one computer unit to another to transmit and receive information.

Compiler. After a computer programmer writes the instructions of a computer program in a computer programming language (such as COBOL, BASIC, or FORTRAN), a compiler is required to translate those human-readable instructions (called a *source language program* or *source code*) into a form that the computer can actually execute (called *machine language* or *object code*). *See also* Computer Language.

Computer-Human Interface. The collective methods by which humans interact with computer units, including the video screens, pointing devices, and conventions for use of the keyboard. *See also* Windowing.

Computer Interface. A method of transferring blocks of data across the boundaries of computer systems, using software, hardware, or a combination of both.

Computer Language. A computer programming language that is used by people such as computer programmers to write instructions for the computer to execute. *See also* BASIC; COBOL; FORTRAN; Compiler.

Computer Literacy. A term used to refer to people's understanding, tolerance, acceptance of, and skill with computer technology.

Computer Program. A series of instructions written in a computer programming language. The instructions control what the computer is to do. For example, a series of instructions may tell the computer to multiply two numbers together and to print the result on a report. *See also* Computer Language.

Computer Programmer. An individual who writes computer programs. *See also* Programmer/Analyst.

Computer Programming. The process of writing the sequence of instructions in a given computer programming language to direct the computer to perform the desired functions. *See also* Computer Language.

Computer System Controls. *See* Software Controls.

Computer Terminal. A video display unit, computer printer, or other input or output device that is used by a person to interact with a computer system. *See also* Video Display Unit.

Controls and Control Processes. Procedures, special forms, approved steps, exception reports, and other measures to prevent, detect, and possibly even correct errors. *See also* Software Controls.

Conversion. The process of transforming data records from a manual or computerized record-keeping process to the computer information system that is replacing it.

Cooperative Processing. A function of distributed processing whereby two or more programs share in the processing of a transaction. Also referred to as client/server processing, in which case one of the computers is called the client and the other, the server. *See also* Distributed Processing.

CPU. *See* Central Processing Unit.

CRT. *See* Cathode Ray Tube.

Data Base. A collection of data files that contains all the data elements retrievable for data analysis.

Data Base Administrator (DBA). An individual responsible for the design, development, operation, safeguarding, and maintenance of a data base.

Data Dictionary. Lists of data elements available for retrieval and analysis, such as in decision support systems or executive information systems. *See also* Data Base.

Data Element (or Data Field). An element of data within a data record, constituting an item of information. For example, patient name, street address, service code, and total price are four data elements. *See also* Data Record; Data File.

Data File. A set of related data records. For example, all the data records of all patients to be billed for service would likely be stored in a computer system as one data file. *See also* Data Element; Data Record.

Data Record. A set of related data elements. For example, all the data elements collected during a patient registration would likely be stored in a computer system as one data record. *See also* Data File; Data Element.

Debug. To detect, diagnose, and eliminate errors in computer programs. *See also* Bug; Acceptance Test; Parallel Test.

Decision Support System (DSS). A data base and data access language by which management and staff may obtain current information for management planning and control.

Default. An option that is assumed when none is explicitly specified.

Desktop Computer. A computer, such as a personal computer, that is designed to be placed, together with optional units, on the top of a desk or table.

Desktop Workstation. *See* Intelligent Workstation.

Direct Access. The ability to retrieve a data record from a storage device, or to enter a data record into a storage device, without being concerned about its specific sequential position relative to other records in the same data file. *Contrast with* Sequential Access.

Disk. A type of computer data storage using spinning circular platters. Data are recorded or retrieved by inserting the disk into a disk drive, which contains a reading and writing device (called a *read/write head*) that moves over the spinning disk.

Disk Drive. A data storage device that houses rotating circular platters (disks). *See also* Disk; Diskette.

Diskette. A flexible data storage disk enclosed in a protective container. Synonymous with floppy disk.

Disk Operating System. *See* DOS.

Disk Storage Unit. *See* Disk; Disk Drive.

Distributed Processing. An information systems strategy in which the computer processing work load is dispersed among computers that are located in different locations throughout the institution. *See also* Cooperative Processing.

DOS (Disk Operating System). Operating system software for an IBM PC and for personal computers that are compatible with the IBM PC.

Dot Matrix Printer. *See* Matrix Printer.

Down. Pertaining to a computer system that is inoperative.

Download. To transfer data from a computer processing unit to a smaller attached device such as a microcomputer for processing. *Contrast with* Upload.

Edit. Used as both a noun and verb, and applies to preventing entry of data that are incorrect. As a noun: the term encompasses a wide range of checks of data accuracy, including checks of presence, format, completeness, and reasonableness. As a verb: to apply an edit. *See also* Software Controls.

End-User Computing. Comprehensive computer usage by someone other than a computer professional, usually involving retrieval and analysis of data. *See also* Decision Support System; Executive Information System.

Ergonomics. Concern for the working environment in which computer systems are used, including the design and color of the video display unit screen, touch and feel of the keyboard, pointing devices, and even the work surface and seating used.

Executive Information System (EIS). An information system individualized to each executive, designed to give executives easy direct access to information, especially the critical indicators of performance that are individually identified by those executives as being important. The system should also allow for extended analysis beyond those indicators when necessary. *See also* Decision Support System.

Executive Support System (ESS). *See* Executive Information System.

Expert System. A computer system that combines access to data and systematic use of stored logic rules to draw inferences and mimic the reasoning of experts. Synonymous with knowledge-based system. *See also* Artificial Intelligence.

Fiber Optics. Strands of glass fibers used to transmit digital data. *Contrast with* Coaxial Cable.

Field. *See* Data Element.

File. *See* Data File.

Floppy Disk. *See* Diskette.

FORTRAN. An early programming language abbreviated from the words *Formula Translator,* and used primarily by mathematical and scientific computer users. The instructions of this language resemble mathematical formulas. *See also* Computer Language.

Fourth-Generation Language (4GL). A computer language considered to be very easy to use, especially for those who are not computer professionals. Languages with this characteristic have begun to come into use fairly recently, after three generations of languages that were not easy to use. *See also* Computer Language; End-User Computing.

Gateway. A functional unit that connects two computer networks of different network architectures. *See also* Network Bridge.

Hard Copy. A printed copy of computer output, such as printed reports.

Hard Disk. A disk storage unit in which the rotating disk cannot be removed, unlike, for example, a diskette. *See also* Disk; Disk Drive.

Hardware. The computer equipment, as opposed to the computer software, of a computer system. *Contrast with* Software.

Hierarchical Data Base. A data base in which the stored data are organized in the form of a tree structure where each data record is subordinate to another, and which predetermines the access paths to data stored in the data base. *Contrast with* Relational Data Base.

Host Computer. In a computer network, the computer that serves other computers as a hub for services, as a source of data, and for other computer processing purposes. *See also* Mainframe.

Image Processing. Processing of digital images, in which the images are represented as a series of ones and zeros each representing the level of light intensity on the surface of the image. Millions of data bits are required to represent information in this manner, requiring high-capacity data storage and high-speed data communications. Diagnostic images are represented in this manner, as will be other patient chart data that must be stored in image form, as opposed to transcribed text form.

Information Center. A responsibility in an information services department, in which one or more employees, fluent in end-user computing languages and decision support systems, are specifically assigned to advise, guide, teach, and offer one-on-one assistance to computer users.

Infrastructure. Sometimes called the *architecture,* or *underlying technology,* the infrastructure includes the hardware and software technology underlying the institution's computer systems.

Intelligent Workstation (or Intelligent Terminal). A desktop computer unit capable of computer processing independent of the main computer system.

Interface. *See* Computer Interface; Computer-Human Interface.

Knowledge-Based System. *See* Expert System.

LAN. *See* Local Area Network.

Laser Printer. A printer that uses a laser beam to create images on paper. *Contrast with* Matrix Printer.

Life Cycle. A life cycle of a computer system is the time during which the system is a viable product in its market. Computer systems are easily displaced by later systems that use newer, more reliable, cheaper, and better technology. The life cycle includes the period of design, development, availability, and, finally, obsolescence.

Light Pen. A light-sensitive pointing device that is used to select system options from a menu presented on a video display unit. The selection is made by simply pointing the light pen at the display surface. *See also* Menu; Computer-Human Interface.

Local Area Network (LAN). A computer network capable of sharing data among computers within an organization or over a local area, usually a single building. *See also* Backbone Network.

Log. A data file in which the computer system automatically stores data records about occurrences of transactions, usually for accounting, backup and recovery, data security, or other auditing purposes. *See also* Audit Trail.

Magnetic Tape. A computer storage medium that makes use of a reel of tape with a magnetizable surface layer on which data are stored by magnetic recording.

Mainframe. A large computer, in particular one to which other computers can be connected so that they can share facilities that the mainframe provides. *See also* Host Computer.

Maintenance. Work performed to support the continued operation of a computer system. Both hardware and software maintenance are periodically required to keep a computer system functioning. *See also* Preventive Maintenance.

Matrix Printer. A printer that prints characters on paper by representing each character as a fairly dense pattern of dots. *Contrast with* Laser Printer.

Megabytes (MB). A measure of the storage capacity of the internal storage or disk storage of a computer system. One megabyte of storage is approximately 1 million bytes, although technically it represents a storage capacity of 2^{20} (1,048,576) bytes. *See also* Byte; Character.

Menu. A list of options, displayed on a CRT screen, to allow a user to select the function to be performed. Computer systems that use menus are called *menu driven*. *See also* Light Pen; Mouse.

Microcomputer. A small computer that can execute computer instructions, such as a personal computer.

Minicomputer. An intermediate-size computer that can perform the same kinds of applications as a mainframe computer but has less storage capacity and processing power than a mainframe.

Modem. A device for changing text and data into a signal that can be transmitted over telephone lines, or the reverse. Derived from the words modulate/demodulate.

Monitor. *See* Video Display Unit.

Mouse. A hand-held device, moved on a flat surface, for selecting from a menu of system options.

Multiprogramming. A mode of computer operation that provides for processing multiple computing tasks simultaneously.

Multitasking. *See* Multiprogramming.

Network Bridge. A functional unit of hardware and software that is used to interconnect two computer networks of similar network architectures. *See also* Gateway.

On-Line. A mode of usage of a computer system that allows users remote from the computer system to access the computer through individual video display units.

Operating System. A set of complex computer programs, normally provided by the hardware vendor, that schedule and manage the computer system's internal processing, including allocating and managing the computer's internal and disk storage, accepting input from the keyboard and other input devices, directing output to video display units, printers, and other devices, and detecting and correcting internal malfunctions. *See also* DOS.

Optical Disk Storage. Data storage technology in which data are stored and read via a laser beam rather than magnetically. *See also* Disk.

Packaged Software. Computer software, marketed by many vendors, designed to be general enough to fulfill the information needs of many institutions. Examples include general ledger systems, accounts payable systems, and accounts receivable systems. *See also* Application Software.

Parallel Test. The method by which the processing of a new computer information system is tested for a period of time against the results of an existing manual or old computer system, using the same input data, to verify that the new system is producing the correct results. *See also* Acceptance Test.

Password. A code of letters, numbers, or both, known only to the authorized user of that password, that is entered into a computer system to gain access.

Performance Management (of Hardware and Software). Procedures, computerized logs, and reports that are used to monitor the utilization, response time, and internal processing of a computer system, in order to sense internal work bottlenecks and performance problems.

Periodic Audit. Procedures undertaken periodically to verify that procedures and computer processing are as they are intended and meet accepted standards of practice of the industry and of the institution. *See also* Audit.

Peripheral Equipment. Components of computer hardware other than the central processing unit and internal memory, such as disk storage units, printing equipment, and equipment used to interconnect the computer to networks and to video display units.

Port. A connection point on a computer or other computer hardware, to which cable connections from video display units, printers, and other data communications devices may be connected.

Portability. The ability to transfer the processing of computer software to a computer of a different mode without modifying the software.

Preventive Maintenance. Scheduled maintenance of computer hardware so as to prevent its failure during operation. *See also* Maintenance.

Problem Management. Systematic recording of problems with computer systems, assignment of priorities and responsibility for remedies, tracking of status, and assessment of frequencies by type of problem, system, and user function, so that long-term plans may be fashioned to prevent frequent reoccurrence.

Program. *See* Computer Program.

Program Libraries. The organized and stored collection of the computer programs of the institution.

Programmer. *See* Computer Programmer.

Programmer/Analyst. A person who performs the combined functions of a programmer and systems analyst. *See also* Computer Programmer; Systems Analyst.

Programming. *See* Computer Programming.

Programming Language. *See* Computer Language.

Project Leader. *See* Project Manager.

Project Manager. A project team member who takes responsibility for leading a project team to ensure that objectives are defined and understood, agreements and approvals are obtained, activities are assigned and scheduled, meetings are scheduled and controlled, minutes of meetings are available, and that other communication occurs among team members and other appropriate people.

Project Team. The team of participants from diverse departments charged with the responsibility for a computer system project, usually led by a project manager or project leader.

Prompt. A symbol or message that is displayed on a video display unit by a computer system to request input from the user.

Protocol. A convention used for data communication between computers, including all the rules for initiating transmission, synchronizing the sending and receiving of transmissions, and detecting and correcting errors in transmissions.

Random Access Memory (RAM). A computer storage device into which data can be entered and retrieved.

Read-Only Memory (ROM). Internal computer memory in which data can be stored once, and cannot be modified thereafter.

Read-Only-Storage. *See* Read-Only Memory.

Recovery. The resetting of the files of a computer system to a previous processing step from which computer processing can be restored and continued without error in functional processing. Recovery usually requires restoring data from a backup copy. *See also* Backup Copy.

Relational Data Base. A data base in which the stored data are organized with cross-references among data elements so that data relationships are represented in the data base. For example, a relational data base may cross-reference all the patients admitted by the same physician. *Contrast with* Hierarchical Data Base.

Response Time. Waiting time experienced at a video display unit after depressing the ENTER key, or other means of requesting work from the computer system, and the response by the computer system. Usually measured in seconds or fractions of seconds.

RISC. An acronym for Reduced Instruction Set Computing, which is electronic computer technology that allows vendors to manufacture powerful computers at reduced cost.

ROM. *See* Read-Only Memory.

Sequential Access. A method of accessing computer data records in which the records are read from, or written to, a data file based on the logical order of the records in the file. *Contrast with* Direct Access.

Server. On a local area network, a computer that provides services to other computers, for example, a file server or a print server.

Software. Computer programs. *Contrast with* Hardware.

Software Controls. Programmed controls in a computer system to detect, and possibly to correct, errors. *See also* Edit.

Software Engineering. A relatively new professional field concerned with timely implementation of reliable software and successful management of its use.

Software Maintenance. *See* Maintenance.

Software Package. *See* Packaged Software.

Source Code. *See* Compiler.

Source Program. *See* Compiler.

Spreadsheet Software. Software that provides the ability to easily process rows and columns of data, automatically calculating totals of values in rows and columns, much as an accountant does in preparing financial reports.

Stand-Alone Computer System. A computer system that is independent of other computer systems, and especially independent of the main computer systems of an institution.

Steering Committee. A group of high-level executives who plan and prioritize computer systems projects for their institution, and monitor and control their implementation progress.

Suspense File. A file containing unprocessed or partially processed items awaiting further action.

Synchronous. Data communication among computers in which the communication is time synchronized, and each character transmitted is expected at the other end within a precise time interval. *Contrast with* Asynchronous.

Systems Analysis. The systematic investigation of a work process to determine how it might be improved, especially with computer automation.

Systems Analyst. A person responsible for investigating work processes and defining the step-by-step processes, especially for the purpose of automating the process using computer technology.

System Design. Defining the data records, data files, and computer programs that would be necessary to automate a work process.

Tape Drive. A magnetic tape recording and reading device into which magnetic tapes are inserted for the storage or retrieval of data. *See also* Magnetic Tape.

Technical Support. Members of a computer systems department who have the responsibility for planning, implementing, and maintaining the operating system software and related technology for networking and data communications. *See also* Operating System.

Technical Plan. A list of activities necessary to plan and develop the technological infrastructure, including technological work activities for up to approximately two years.

Teleprocessing. The means of providing data communication links among computers. *See also* Communication Link.

Terminal. *See* Computer Terminal.

Testing. *See* Debug; Acceptance Test; Parallel Test.

Token Passing. In a token ring network, the process by which the many computers take turns using a local area network. *See also* Token Ring Network.

Token Ring Network. A local area network among computers, configured as a closed ring, and in which token passing is the means of forcing the computers to take turns using the network. *See also* Token Passing; Local Area Network.

Touch Screen. A visual display unit that has a screen that is sensitive to touch, and through which menu options are chosen by touching the screen directly over the desired option. *See also* Menu; User Friendly; Computer-Human Interface. *Contrast with* Light Pen; Mouse.

Transaction. One unit of computerized work, usually requested by a user at a video display unit, to accomplish a particular result, such as the registration of a patient.

Transaction Logging. *See* Log.

Transaction Trail. *See* Audit Trail.

Turn-Key System. A computer system supplied by a vendor to a customer in a ready-to-run condition, requiring little or no preparatory work by the customer.

Uninterruptible Power Supply (UPS). An emergency source of electrical power that is available and ready to be drawn into use in the event that the normal source of electrical power fails for a short period of time.

UNIX. An operating system that can be used in mainframe computers, minicomputers, as well as microcomputers. It includes comprehensive multitasking capabilities that personal microcomputer operating systems such as DOS do not. UNIX is available from AT&T, its developer, but there are also several variations available, some known also as UNIX, some known by other names, such as AIX from IBM. *See also* Operating System; DOS.

Upload. To transfer data from a small computer such as a personal computer, to a large computer. *Contrast with* Download.

UPS. *See* Uninterruptible Power Supply.

User Friendly. The characteristic of a computer information system that makes it easy to use by people who are not computer professionals. *See also* Computer-Human Interface.

User Inquiry Language. A user language that allows the direct presentation of analytical and summary data on the video terminal, on printers nearby, or both. This concept is included in decision support systems. *See also* Decision Support Systems.

User Interface. *See* Computer-Human Interface.

Video Display Unit (VDU). A device with a TV-like display screen, usually equipped with a keyboard. Synonymous with video display terminal, visual display unit, visual display terminal, monitors, and cathode ray tube.

Visual Display Unit. *See* Video Display Unit.

Windowing. A strategy for making computer systems easy to use by displaying information on a video display unit in what appear to be windows, dividing a display screen into sections that can be simultaneously displayed. *See also* Computer-Human Interface; User Friendly.

Wiring Closet. A room that contains one or more equipment racks and distribution panels that are used to connect cables from computers to a network or to each other.

INDEX

ABOUT THE AUTHOR

Bernie Minard is Senior Vice President of The Methodist Hospital, a 1527-bed teaching hospital for Baylor College of Medicine. Methodist is the largest private hospital in the United States, and one of the premier facilities of the Texas Medical Center in Houston. As an executive at Methodist since 1980, Mr. Minard has led its computer technology activities and has been a member of a senior management team that has won national acclaim. In 1989, the hospital received the *Healthcare Forum*/Witt Associates Commitment to Quality Award and was recognized by *Healthcare Forum* as one of the ten most successful hospitals in the United States. In 1990, *BusinessWeek* recognized the hospital as one of the best-run nonprofit health care organizations in the United States. In 1991, it received the Shared Data Research Award of Excellence for hospitals with the best overall information systems.

Mr. Minard earned his M.S. in statistics at Stanford University and his bachelor's degree in electrical engineering at the University of Louisville. His background includes assignments in computer systems management in support of the NASA program, as well as management assignments for a multinational energy company, including the establishment of a computer center and computer systems department in Europe. He has published articles in a number of periodicals, including *Hospital & Health Services Administration, Healthcare Financial Management, Computers in Healthcare, Healthcare Informatics, CIO, HealthTexas,* and *Healthcare Strategic Management.* He has served as a board member or officer of many industry groups, including the Houston Chapter of the Society for Information Management, the Texas Hospital Association Information Systems Society, the Houston Chapter of the Hospital Information and Management Systems Society (HIMSS), and the Texas State Technical Institute Computer Science Advisory Board. In addition, he is a member of several industry committees, including the Texas Hospital Association Data Management Committee and the Rice University Graduate School of Business Committee on Management of Information Technology. He is a member of the American College of Healthcare Executives.